FITNESS OVER 40

BUILD MORE MUSCLE, STRENGTH & AGILITY WHILE SUPERCHARGING YOUR HEALTH AS A 40, 50 OR 60+ YEAR OLD USING THESE STRENGTH TRAINING EXERCISES & NUTRITION GUIDES

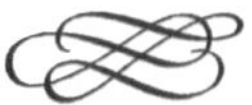

FEMI EMMA

CONTENTS

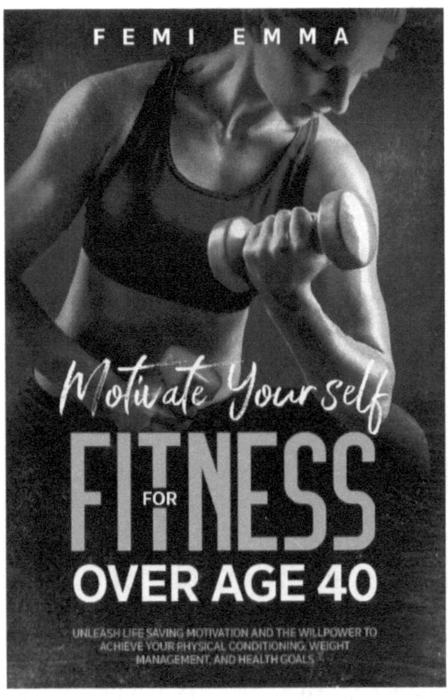

If you are over the age of 40 and believe in the importance of exercising and getting into shape but can't seem to fire up your motivation and willpower to *start working out*, this is the one book you need to read now. Ask yourself these questions:

- Do you believe you should take exercise seriously, especially after the age of 40, when things start slowing down and new physical issues start showing up?

- Are you impressed when you see someone lifting
  weights, doing push-ups, or pulling cables on a
  resistance machine and wish you could get stronger
  with bigger muscles?
- When you see others jogging, walking, swimming,
  biking, or working out on elliptical machines, do you
  say to yourself, "I should be doing cardiovascular
  conditioning for my heart?"

A 'yes' answer to any or all of these questions means you
know you should get going with an exercise routine but just
haven't ignited the spark or kept it burning. It's all about motivation and willpower, and this book will:

- Ignite your motivation with compelling reasons *why*
  to deeply commit to exercise and fitness.
- Give you the *willpower* and resolve to get started now
  and make exercise an essential part of your life.
- Inspire you to follow a holistic, healthy lifestyle of
  responsible exercise and diet.

Hundreds of others are already enjoying insider access to all
of my current future books. If you want insider access plus
this Fitness Book, all you have to do is **scan the code** below
with your smartphone camera to claim your offer.

Don't hesitate! This amazing book can be yours today if you take advantage of this free offer. We respect your privacy, so your email address will be kept safe and will not be sold or shared with others.

INTRODUCTION

I know firsthand that strength, muscle, and fitness can come to anyone, at any age. After all, I started gaining muscle "late"— I took up strength training in my 30s, and by the time I'd reached my 40s, I was already enjoying the clear and profound results.

I'm nobody special; I'm the perfect example of how an untalented, ungifted, and relatively normal person can get into great shape. The only thing I've ever had going for me was that I found strength training really interesting—when I got into strength and muscle training, I seriously nerded out on every book, article, and video I could get my hands on.

The truth is a simple and beautiful one: **If you do it right, there's no reason you can't get into the best shape of your life in your 40s and beyond**. Especially if you're new to strength training, you can achieve fantastic results that are *so often ignored* when people talk about fitness over 40.

It doesn't all need to be salads, kale, quinoa, and endurance. You can do more than get in shape; you can get strong, you can build muscle, and you can look like the most athletic, outstanding, confident version of yourself. The only thing holding you back has been the expectations other people have of you—perhaps the ones you've had for yourself—and lacking the information and guidance you need to put it all into action.

I've worked with this exact kind of mindset, as a personal trainer and over-40s strength specialist, for over a decade. It's my own experience—getting into the shape of my life and building muscle over 40—and I can tell you that I have hundreds (if not thousands) of successful client stories that back up this exact same transformation process.

I often look back on the worries and expectations I used to have and feel like I could have started sooner if I'd just known what I was doing, and if I'd known that I **could** make an amazing physical change. That's why I've written this book: I want you to have the knowledge and experience I've gained by *doing* over the past 15 years, from nutrition to training to recovery.

INSTRUCTIONS: HOW TO USE THIS BOOK

Let's be real here—we already start to age from the moment we are conceived. The fact is, aging is not an evil to be overcome. Actually, it can be quite pleasant! But when it comes to physical activity, preconceptions affect our motivation to move. The processes associated with aging, such as chronic conditions, diabetes, elevated blood pressure, arthritis, and back problems—to name but a few—are actually very similar to the ones induced by physical inactivity. The reality is that the symptoms of 'aging' could actually be re-labelled as symptoms of 'disuse' (Bortz, "Disuse and Aging", *Journal of the American Medical Association*).

If this is not evidence enough, additional scientific and medical evidence should motivate you to get moving. Dr. Dorothy V. Harris and Dr. Bette L. Harris provide many more reasons to be physically active: "Exercise is nature's best tranquilizer" (*The Athlete's Guide to Sports Psychology: Mental Skills for Physical People*) because it boosts serotonin levels in the brain. Researchers have found that individuals suffering from moderate to light depression who regularly engage in at least 15 to 30 minutes of aerobic exercise typically experience an improvement in their condition.

This book will give you the tools to understand how you should be moving, either at home or in an equipped gym. All you should know about the physiology happening when you use your muscles, as well as how to treat them well and help them heal, will be explained in this book. Your posture is something that needs to be addressed, too: this is the foundation of all workouts! Identifying which body type you are will also provide you with customized tips on how to become fit accordingly.

Different workouts are explained—strength training and cardio training, and their variations, from HIIT (High Intensity Interval Training) to weightlifting. These are all good, but they require to be set up, following a pattern and a schedule according to specific factors. Do not fret. This book suggests a training plan that you can tailor to yourself, modifying the weight you can work out with (either body weight or added resistance of dumbbells). The different positions and exercises are all explained using visual aids. The muscles these exercises target are detailed in illustrations that I call 'Muscle

Maps', as well as the reasons to avoid specific positions. I will give you the keys in this book to adapt these workouts for you and your body. Following the visuals and the explanations will help you avoid injury.

As good health starts inward, it is important that you understand the basics of nutrition and how to adapt it to your body type. First, we need to address the issue of calories and abandon the idea of fad diets. In your 40s and beyond, you have to be careful not to attempt to 'lose weight' at all costs—this can lead you to lose muscle mass as well as water, even if it is not intended.

Let's actually talk about wanting to lose fat or gain muscle mass. Your goal has a real impact on how you should be eating. For both, your food and liquids intake needs to be pretty balanced and combine most—or all, ideally—vitamins and minerals required. People with chronic conditions, whether epilepsy, diabetes, elevated blood pressure or recovering from a previous surgery—at any age—will benefit from a specialist's knowledge and a personalized diet and fitness plan.

Aids are given in this book for you to assess and track your progress. You are obviously already motivated, as you've picked up this book and gotten this far! Now, let me share with you my knowledge to stay or become fit after 40, and let's do this together.

Dr. Bortz said in his book, _We Live Too Short and Die Too Long_, "We now know that a very fit body of 70 can be the same as a moderately fit body of 30." Let's start today together to be as active as when we were 30.

*"It's going to be a **JOURNEY**. It's not a sprint to get in shape."*

— KERRI WALSH JENNINGS

PART I
GETTING TO PROPERLY KNOW YOUR BODY

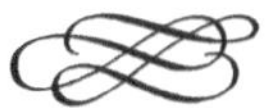

You are your body, but you probably don't know it as well as you should. After all, it doesn't come with a user manual, and the education system doesn't place much focus on teaching you how to take care of it!

To get the most out of strength training, you need to build a better—and more understanding—relationship with your body. Let's take a quick look at how the body works and how you can make it work for you, in the pursuit of improved strength, health, and fitness.

MISCONCEPTIONS AROUND AGING, MUSCLE AND STRENGTH TRAINING

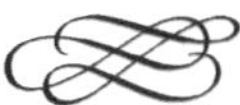

There are a lot of incorrect ideas floating around when it comes to aging and strength training—the conceptions people have about how we age and what it does to the body are, often, **simply wrong**.

The classic idea of aging gracefully—of not doing any exercise and resigning yourself to a steady decline—is well out of fashion. Rather, we're seeing the science suggest the opposite: you only decline if you let these expectations stop you from doing healthy exercise or eating in a considered way.

The way that over-40s are portrayed in media definitely contributes to this: the expectation of aging and decline is one of the causes of it! **Changes in behavior are the problem, not changes in age**.

THE WAY OVER 40S ARE PAINTED IN THE MEDIA

Everywhere you look, you're going to see people aging badly —almost like it's inevitable. The way we treat life after 40 is steadily becoming more reasonable, but for generations it's been the "midlife" stage where we are all meant to put on our comfy slippers and start taking it easy.

As nice as it sounds, that's not how the body works, and it's not reflective of how fit, healthy, and active we can all be for a whole lifetime. The expectation produces the problem, and not the other way around: *you don't stop lifting weights because you age, you age because you stop lifting weights.*

The things that make you feel strong, healthy, and confident in your 20s are the same in your 40s, 60s, and 80s. You might need to undo a few decades of bad habits along the way, but you're also armed with the wisdom and patience of experience!

Kicking off the comfy slippers and getting or staying active means holding off the worst effects of aging but, even more than that, you can continue to improve well into and beyond your 40s. Unless you were an elite athlete in your younger years, there's no reason you can't get into the shape of your life **now**.

Expectations only change when we prove them wrong: strength training over 40 is growing and setting new standards, and the old stereotypes of exercise after 40 are evolving beyond golf and yoga. Strength suits you at all ages, and the science tells us it's only more important as we get older.

EXPECTATIONS DRIVE DECLINE, NOT THE OTHER WAY AROUND

I mentioned this above, but there is no necessity to getting old, pudgy, and inactive. The changes that happen to diet, sleep, and exercise are the main drivers to these changes—and they're far from unavoidable.

Hell, you wouldn't be reading this book if you were resigned to this kind of lifestyle!

There are changes that happen in the body as we age, but we're not stuck with them. If you pick up exercise at 40 after decades of inactivity, you'll have better hormonal health and improved strength compared to what you experienced in your 20s.

This is because **behaviors dictate the body's health and performance**, rather than the other way around. The problems of aging are associated with dropping crucial habits that strengthen and maintain the body—the effects of aging only lead to decline *if you're already in perfect shape.*

If we keep up these crucial behaviors, then the result is not only maintenance, but progress. We can see this with all kinds of elite athletes and sportspeople: there are a handful of Olympians over 40, while we see martial artists like the Gracies practice jiu-jitsu into their **nineties**.

Sport, exercise, and activity keep us young—and our health and fitness only change after 40 if we forget the joy of movement and the confidence of strength.

A YEAR IS NOT THE SAME FOR EVERYONE

One of the things we learn from other cultures is that the way we treat age is weird—closely tying together age and expectations of health and strength doesn't make a lot of sense.

There is not a single effect of a year on your health. The way we age—the changes a year produces—are completely individual, based on the ways that we live. Forty years is completely different for someone smoking, drinking, and binge-eating compared to someone living a healthy and active lifestyle, full of exercise, lean proteins, and veggies.

The number of years under your belt doesn't determine your health, it's a function: it multiplies your habits. Imagine the effect of 40 years of bad habits, but also imagine 50 years of good ones—who is likely to be doing better?

This is the choice we have before us, and it's important to make sure that the years to come will build good habits and positive change.

STRENGTH GETS MORE IMPORTANT AS WE AGE

There **are** conditions we have to guard ourselves against as our age increases, such as osteoporosis, metabolic syndrome, and fractures. These are a part of getting older, but the problem is that we use them as an excuse to be inactive and hide away from the possibility of injury through exercise.

This is completely wrong: strength is **more** important as we age, since maintaining what we've got and building additional strength, muscle, and fitness staves off these problems. It's also harder to succumb to frailty when you've got a surplus. If you're losing a pound of muscle a year from aging, having 10 extra pounds of muscle means 10 more good years in the bank!

This is the *medical* reason for strength training over 40. It reduces the risk of any changes to the body, as well as buying you even better, healthy, active years down the road. If you're in your 40s or 50s, the work you do now isn't just going to mean looking and feeling great this year, but also building another decade of quality living into your 80s, for example.

You can still reach amazing goals in your 40s, 50s and beyond with proper habits, and it's clear that your body doesn't **need** to fall apart—it's all down to what you choose to do and how you use your body. That's why we need to talk about how your body works, and how you can get it to work for you…

HOW YOUR BODY WORKS — A USER'S GUIDE

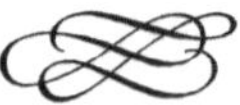

*Y*our body didn't come with an owner's manual, so I'm going to catch you up to speed on the most important processes. These are important for health and fitness, but they're also a great insight into how you work and how you should be structuring your life.

I'm obviously only going to cover these briefly, because the human body is a complicated thing and there's more biology than I could ever fit into one book. What matters are the **principles**: the things we know about the body that help us understand what to do with it!

BASICS OF ANATOMY

The 'muscle maps' below highlights the main muscles, showing both the front and the back views. Use this chart to identify which muscles are targeted during the workouts.

Wolff's law states that the strength of a bone is directly correlated to the force applied to it. This is due to the bone bearing more weight by targeting the attached muscles. Thus, strength training increases bone density significantly—a beneficial factor to consider when aging, especially as a woman.

The only way to grow muscle tissue is to injure the muscle by challenging its fibers. Neighboring cells are directed on the muscle tear, fusing together and causing muscle growth. This is a microscopic growth, so you need to do this repeatedly.

When exercised, the muscle generates lactic acid, or lactate, which causes a burning feeling but subsides during the resting period. This "burn" indicates that the muscle needs some rest: take a short break and then continue. Gradually, the burn will intervene later in your workout and after more reps.

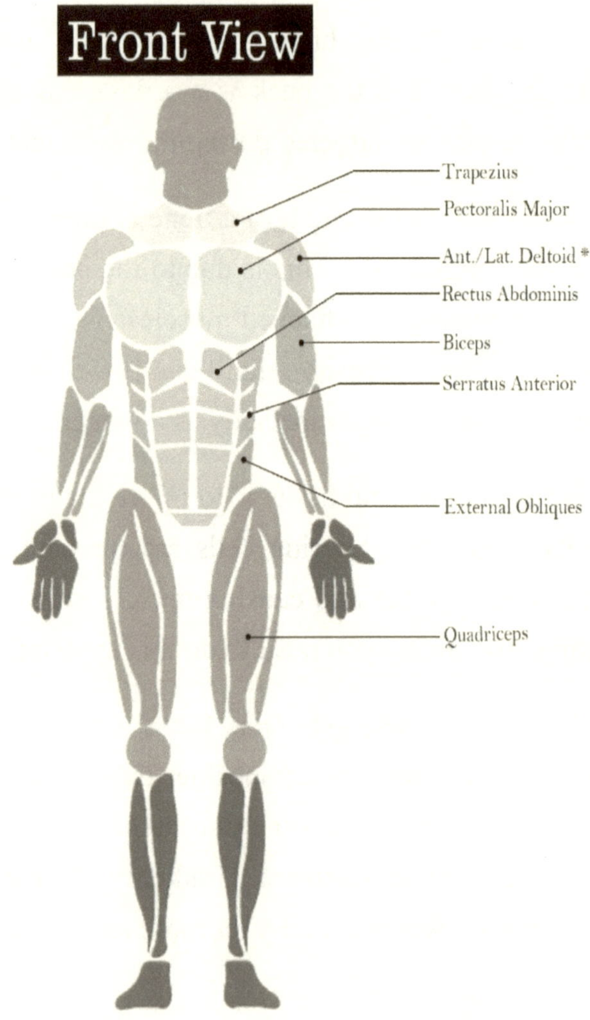

Ant./Lat. Deltoid – Anterior/Lateral Deltoid, as specified in Strength Training Exercises chapter.

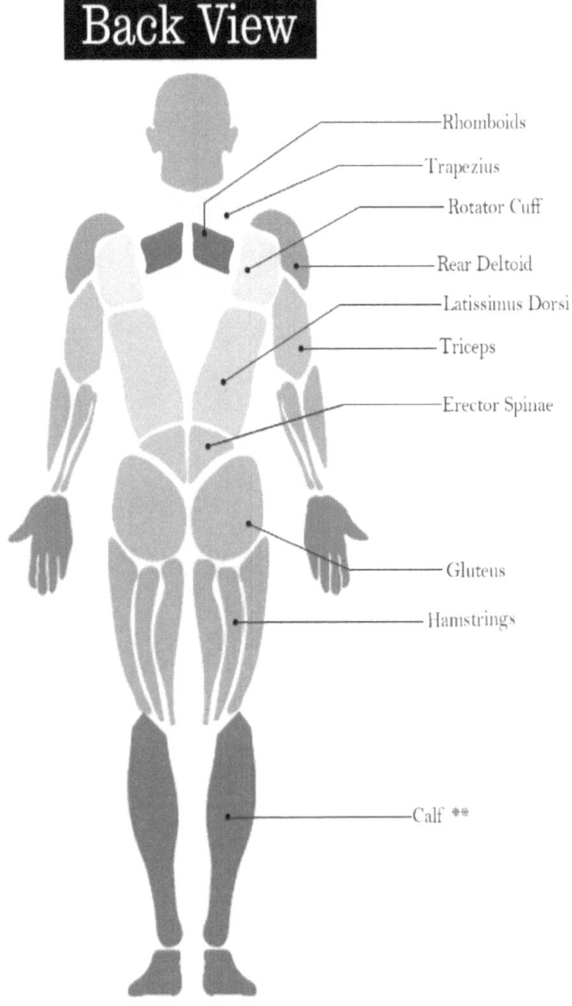

*** Calf – Soleus/Gastrocnemius as specified in Strength Training
Exercises chapter.*

After a workout, increased soreness, or no soreness at all, doesn't necessarily mean you did too much or not enough. Muscles can react differently to the same training, for no apparent reason. Sometimes,

pain called Delayed Onset Muscle Soreness (DOMS) appears later, associated as much with the strain put on the muscle as to the muscle cells regenerating. This is good pain!

UNDERSTANDING YOUR BODY

The way your body looks is a result of your genetics combined with environmental factors including nutrition and training. These are factors that you can consciously change and alter every day. However, the genetic factor, which has a dominant influence on your body structure as well as the prenatal development, is an element you cannot change.

WHAT ARE BODY TYPES?

Body types were defined in the 1940s by American doctor W.H. Sheldon. You can, by knowing yourself, determine your body type. If you wish to find the exact ponderation of your body type as defined by Sheldon, websites will do the calculation for you. Your body type will determine the workout routine and diet plan that will work best for you.

HOW DO YOU IDENTIFY YOUR OWN BODY TYPE?

In order to determine your body type, you'll have to look critically at your body, your past weight, and muscle journey. This will allow you to identify the main body type you are—either a dominant ectomorph, a dominant mesomorph, or a dominant endomorph. Then, you can adapt your training and nutritional journey accordingly.

Typically, the **ectomorph** is a person who struggles to gain either fat or muscle, having a naturally slim build—lean, as we would say nowadays. The tall and very thin Ethiopian runners are the extreme of this body shape.

A **mesomorph** body is 'average,' without being disparaging in any way. Their build is not especially large or muscular, nor round and fat. For the mesomorph, it is easy to gain muscle, but also fat if inactive.

Endomorph people have to pay close attention to their food intake and add a certain amount of cardio to reduce their fat proportion. Indeed, they tend to be more fat, with some belly, double chins, and wide hips for women. Do not despair, as this type can also add muscle easily, but has to monitor their diet carefully.

There are rules to follow common to all body types:

- Always warm up all muscles and stretch lightly before picking up any weights.
- Employ split-training: working one or two body parts during each workout to target muscle groups.
- Train each body part twice a week, if possible.
- Work your core muscles three times per week, 3 sets of 25 of two different exercises (e.g. crunches and leg lifts).
- Get plenty of rest between workouts.
- Don't train if your body part is still sore from a previous workout. Increase training intensity slowly to avoid strain or injury.
- Good cardio exercises include using the elliptical machine, the stationary bike, and the treadmill, or running, biking, and brisk walking.
- Your daily protein intake should be 1 to 1.6 grams of protein per kilo of body weight (Gastelu and Hatfield 2019). It should amount to 30% of your daily intake, with 50% carbohydrates, and 20% fats. This is further explained in the nutrition chapter.
- For carbohydrates, increase daily intake of the fibrous type while limiting the intake of simple sugars (e.g. soda, chocolate bars). This is associated with food with a slow-burning glycemic index, such as beans,

corn, sweet potatoes, oats, pasta, brown rice, and whole grain breads.

- Limit or ban alcohol; reduce or stop smoking.
- Finally, drink at least eight 8oz glasses of water per day. Coffee and tea don't count.

The following distinctions appear regarding the way our muscle fibers react, our cardiovascular system works, as well as our energy consumption:

	Ectomorph	Mesomorph	Endomorph
Weight training	Aim for 8 to 10 repetitions per set and do 2 to 3 sets of each exercise.	During split-training, do upper body parts first, then follow with lower body parts.	Aim for 3 sets of no more than 8 repetitions. When you can easily do 8, increase the weight.
	Try different routines and exercises for muscle confusion.	Aim for 3 sets of 8 for each exercise.	Try different routines and exercises for muscle confusion.
	If you stay sore for more than 3 days, you may be lifting too heavy. Scale back on your weight and increase slowly.	Change your workout routine every 2 months by adding new exercises.	Train hard for maximum fat-burning effect while building lean muscle mass.
	If gains in muscle and strength seem stagnant, add weight until you are limited to 8 reps per set.	If gains in muscle and strength seem stagnant, try adding extra weight and one more set to each of your exercises.	

	Ectomorph	Mesomorph	Endomorph
Cardio training	Keep cardio activity to a minimum, no more than 3 times per week, followed by 5 minutes of cool down.	Undertake some cardio activity 3 times per week for 30 minutes, followed by 5 minutes of cool down.	Undertake some cardio activity 3 to 5 times per week for 30 minutes, followed by 5 minutes of cool down.
	Keep cardio conditioning at 70% of your max heart rate for no more than 20 minutes per session.	Keep cardio conditioning at 70% of your max heart rate for no more than 20 minutes per session until you build your cardiovascular system, then you can raise your target heart rate.	Keep cardio conditioning at 70% of your max heart rate for no more than 20 minutes per session until you build your cardiovascular system, then you can raise your target heart rate.
			For added fat burning find a good HIIT (High Intensity Interval Training) program and work into it slowly.

	Ectomorph	Mesomorph	Endomorph
Nutrition	Consume 6 small meals per day.	Consume 5 or 6 small meals per day.	Consume 5 or 6 small meals per day, watching your calorie intake.
	Drink a protein shake after your workout and one at bedtime.	Drink a protein shake mid-morning and after your workout.	Drink a protein shake after your workout and one at bedtime.
		Use low-fat (2%) milk for your protein shakes.	Use non-fat milk or water for your protein shakes.

Knowing this will help you understand the exercises that will help you lose fat and gain muscle, as well as the best way to adapt your nutrition. Crucially, it will also help you plan the long term of your body development. Set yourself up for reasonable goals.

Human physiology, especially associated with aging, is now explored.

BASIC PHYSIOLOGY: HORMONES AND DECLINE

The major concerns that most people have around aging—the things that **do** need to be addressed—are usually hormonal. As we age, the concentrations of key hormones in our bodies are likely to decrease, mildly, year by year. This process starts somewhere around the mid- to late-thirties, and it does undermine some aspects of the body—like how much muscle mass we can hold, a reduction in bone density, and similar effects.

However, what most people don't know is that hormones aren't just a setting in your body on a countdown to frailty. Rather, they're the result of what we do, at least as much as our genetics: hormones affect your life, but they're also dictated by it. The hormonal profile of a sedentary, over-eating, alcoholic 20-year-old smoker is likely to be worse than a 40-year-old with a great strength training routine and a lifestyle to match.

Testosterone is one of the most important hormones for men, while women experience changes in **estrogen** production around their 40s. For medical concerns, consult your doctor—they know you and what you need. For everything else, adopting a healthy lifestyle is a crucial way to rebalance these hormones.

Your hormones respond to your activity level, stress, diet, sleep quality and quantity, as well as your habits like drug and alcohol consumption. If you can control these through lifestyle, then it's clear that you can control the changes in your body—and that's why I say that **behavior** is key to changes in the body, rather than just the number of times you've circled the sun!

BASIC PHYSIOLOGY: THE STRESS-ADAPTATION MODEL (SAM)

The way your body adapts and improves is central to fitness, and strength is the single most obvious example of this. It's called the stress-adaptation model, and it goes like this:

1. You're exposed to a stressor.
2. You recover from that stressor.
3. Your body improves to compensate for possible future stressors.

This is a simple three-step guide to how your body works in a wide variety of areas, from strength to metabolism. The way your body changes is directly linked to the things you do, so your behaviors are crucial to who and what you become in the future.

For fitness, exercise is the stressor, and recovery is built up out of the factors I mentioned above—sleep, diet, hydration, stress levels, and so on. These are important because the better you recover, the more resources you give to step three: improving!

This is going to be a crucial process further into this book when we look at how you should train, how you handle nutrition, and how you progress. In the meantime, just remember that stress-adaptation is what your body does best, and it's the driving force behind getting stronger and fitter.

THE MAIN CHALLENGES OF AGING

As we age, we will face challenges, and it's important to accept this truth. We have to stand up against challenges with good behaviors and hard work—and they pay off when it comes to quality of life, confidence, and longevity.

There are a few I need to highlight, because while they're important by themselves, they're also all closely tied to how we choose to live. They're the main ways that strength and fitness are medically useful, as well as improving the physique and self-confidence.

Sarcopenia

This age-related muscle decline is tied into the testosterone changes mentioned above, but it's also closely related to the onset of inactivity as you age: as you move less, you accelerate the loss of muscle, and thus what movements you *can* do.

Sarcopenia will slowly happen eventually, but it can be postponed by an active lifestyle with strength training and proper nutrition. If you reduce activity as you age, the combination of these two is disastrous, causing muscle to waste away over time.

However, this is only true if you combine these two issues.

If, instead, you're staying active and strength training, your muscles are still able to grow for many years after you're 40. After that, exercise is there to maintain them and preserve them.

Sarcopenia is associated with many other issues like arthritis and chronic joint pain, so it's worth working on sooner rather than later. Bigger, stronger muscles aren't just for show—they're the basis for how we move, so investing in them with your time and effort pays off aesthetically, but also medically.

One of the main areas where this will show is *independent mobility* as you age: in later years, this means being able to walk without assistance, reduced fracture risks, and self-sufficiency. It's not just something to worry about when you're well into your advanced years, though—this kind of combatting starts sooner than you'd think.

Combatting sarcopenia and building muscle can radically reduce the risk of joint injuries all throughout the body. It also helps to regulate the metabolism and control body fat levels, and is one of the most important ways to build power—a crucial anti-injury trait that most people completely ignore.

Hormonal change

I've briefly touched on this, but hormonal changes are complicated. For men, decline in testosterone is a concern because it affects the mind and body. Decreased testosterone means increased sarcopenia risk, but also reductions in confidence, increased problems with mood disorders like depression, and is associated with male suicidality.

For women, changes in estrogen levels during their 40s and 50s are closely related to bone density changes, increased risk of breast cancer. These are also tied to mood disorders, and associated with significant metabolic changes.

Collectively, these changes in the most important hormones range from the body to the mind, from strength to suicidality, and from bone density to depression. It's clear that they need to be considered and—once again—it's important to remember that they're all related to lifestyle and can be protected against with structured, deliberate activity and diet.

Cognitive change

Mental performance and health changes are common during these years, where the hormonal shifts pose risks to the brain. This is also a part of the brain's cycle of breakdown and regeneration, which leans more and more toward breakdown as you age.

Again, we know well that the brain responds to what we do and what we eat. Exercise has long been understood as a factor in keeping the brain healthy, but there are also various nutrients that affect the performance and maintenance of the brain, especially as we age.

For example, a diet rich in omega-3 fats and vitamin D is going to protect the brain and support the regeneration side of the balance. This means reduced cognitive decline—especially if you pair it with regular and appropriate levels of exercise.

Cardiorespiratory health and fitness

The heart does a ton of work over our lifetime and this places it at risk as we age, even at the best of times. This is even more appropriate since the number one cause of death right now is coronary heart disease: a lifestyle-related condition that many people will grapple with. This sits alongside conditions like stroke and acute heart attack as some of the most common natural killers.

Keeping the heart healthy is one of the more obvious aspects of fitness—especially endurance and "cardio" exercise, which is already named after the heart. Of course, lifestyle and diet play a huge factor in heart health, being closely related to the way your heart functions, how well it's maintained, and how hard it has to work to keep up with your diet and habits.

Working on your cardio is important because it prevents the risk of numerous diseases that are already well-known for their prevalence and danger!

Bone density and joint health

The loss of bone mineral density is something we never **see**, unlike sarcopenia, but which affects us all massively. Bones are often thought of as just scaffolding in the body, but they're *alive* and they do a ton of important things that they rarely get credit for, like keeping our blood healthy.

One of the things that occurs as we age is, often, the loss of density in these crucial organs. As this happens, the risk of fractures goes up—both the frequency and the severity, as well as how little it takes to cause them.

The result of this is that many older people can get into cycles of breaks and weakness that leave them in and out of hospital for the last years of their lives. Nobody wants this, especially since bone density is something that responds **really well** to exercise—particularly strength training.

Just like muscles, these crucial tissues get stronger when we stress them—which, again, provides a huge buffer and surplus to combat aging. Equally, preservation of bone mass as we age is related to the hormones mentioned above, as well as the dietary raw materials that we provide for bone regeneration and remodeling.

The combination of the loss of bone density and the loss of muscle mass (sarcopenia) produces significant joint risk. The joints are supported and reinforced by muscle tissues, and reductions make them unstable. Equally, the lowered bone mineral density increases the risk of common medical joint risks like arthritis.

These are compounded by the fact that the tissues connecting muscles to bones—the tendons—are also degrading when we are inactive. These are very slow to build up so, when they're degraded, they can be difficult to repair. Fortunately, regular strength training, good nutrition, and plenty of sleep all help to keep your tendons strong and healthy.

Maintaining these tissues with a healthy lifestyle is key, and strengthening them sooner rather than later massively improves your quality of life. It's an investment that pays off more and more with each passing year, staving off frailty and preventing further joint problems.

The development of a better lifestyle is thus the "secret" to living a long, healthy, happy, and active life without dealing with the musculoskeletal risks we often associate with age.

Quality of life changes

Aside from the various medical benefits, the quality of life returns of exercise and a healthy lifestyle only go up as we age. By the time we're into the 40s and beyond, the difference between working out and *not* doing so is immense for life-style, appearance, and confidence.

These are things that we all look for all the time—they're personal development goals we all hold for ourselves, secretly or openly. Improving the way you look and feel is an amazing investment of your time, and quality of life changes include sexual health, physical performance, increased self-confidence and self-determination, and improved mental well-being.

Something as simple as how energetic you feel plays a huge role in your happiness, and this is just one of the various quality of life changes you can expect from a healthy diet and exercise. Equally, sleep and stress management are improved, which contributes to a healthier and happier life.

Strength training and the associated lifestyle changes are *an upward spiral:* they make things better, and they make it easy to make things better. This is the commitment you're making with this book, and the differences are immense.

GETTING SET FOR TRAINING — PREPARATION AND PROGRESS

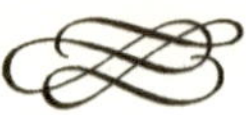

Setting up for fitness is a part of succeeding in strength training. It takes a smart approach to maximize results, and I'm going to explain how you manage that. After all, many people fail with fitness because their approach is wrong, not because they're weak or unmotivated.

Getting it right from the start ensures you're on the right path and that you don't have to double back and try again. This is going to cover a few areas that really need to be set out properly:

- Expectations
- Goal setting
- Setting reasonable timelines
- Appreciating the process (at least) as much as the goal

- Building systems to keep yourself going
- Key factors for training

Each point listed above will teach you a few things about why people fail and how you can avoid this failure. Let's get into them so you can ask yourself key questions: what are **your** goals, how are you going to avoid getting demotivated, and what are you going to do to maximize results from the outset?

EXPECTATIONS: WHY PEOPLE FAIL

One of the main causes of failure is poor expectations. When we get the expectations wrong, disheartenment and disappointment are inevitable – and this is something we see **all the time** when it comes to strength training, especially for the over-40s. Odds are you've experienced this yourself, in the past, and that's why you're reading this book.

Underperforming against our own expectations is a common sight and the problem is that there are two moving parts: performance and expectation. These can both go wrong, but more often we see people who get the expectations wrong— setting the bar too high, then mistakenly thinking their performance was the problem.

Setting expectations is important: we need to be realistic and remember that fitness is a lifelong process and not a short-term solution. How can we fix a lifetime of bad habits in a short time? It's just not possible—and it wouldn't stick if it was!

Set low expectations and be willing to move them up regularly when you meet them. This change of approach is key—and you need to get past "I want to lose 30lbs of fat in the next four weeks" type of goals.

We're adults and we need to be willing to commit to a longer process than that. In fact, timelines themselves are crucial to setting expectations and then goals.

UNDERSTANDING YOUR SUCCESS TIMELINE

Setting your timeline *long* is the key. Short-term changes are fickle and it's no surprise that they're often lost after they're achieved, with 93% of people failing to stick with diets over time. The difference is the amount of success expected and the time given to it.

Your body doesn't do anything that fast—it's a system of slow adaptations to stressors. You need to find a training and exercise routine **you can see yourself doing forever**: that's the timeline of your ultimate strength, health, and fitness goal.

Of course, we can also return to 30lbs of fat loss—a goal that should take roughly half a year. That's a 6-month goal, but the time is going to pass regardless, and during that time there are further benefits like changes to muscle mass, appearance, and confidence.

We need to set longer-term goals that are in line with how the body works. We can achieve shorter-term goals, but our immediate results can't be sustained for months at a time. Short-term results are big, then stall and, when this plateau hits, many people feel like they're failing.

Let's be clear from the start: **losing a pound of fat every seven to ten days is a huge success, as is gaining half a pound of muscle**. That's the pace the normal person's body takes, and that's what you need to set your goals around, rather than rapid fat loss or muscle gain.

This is where you center your expectations: a rate of weight loss or gain that can be sustained over time and helps you keep on track with the goals you're setting—the next step in a successful approach to strength training.

SIMPLE TIERED GOAL-SETTING FOR STRENGTH TRAINING

You need more than one goal, or you're going to fail somewhere along the line. Big goals are too far-off to feel relevant in everyday life, while goals that are too small aren't rewarding and don't motivate us to keep going when things get tough.

Everyone who wants to change their life needs big, medium, and small goals. The big ones are what you want to **be**: athletic, healthy, strong, whatever. It could be that 30lbs of fat loss, regaining strength and aesthetics from youth, or competing in a sport. It just needs to be something that motivates you to keep going for six to 12 months from *today*.

This can be anything you want and as outrageous as you feel like you can achieve, but within the realistic timelines I mentioned above. The key here is that it's not the **only** goal you're relying on, so you can avoid feeling like you've failed while you're on the journey.

Medium goals should be something you work toward where you can see direct progress. Humans need a sense of meaningful progression to really feel like we're doing something useful and maintain motivation.

Medium goals can be anything that you want to achieve in the next two to six weeks. It could be your next size down, your next 10lbs milestone, or the next 10kg on an exercise you really enjoy or benefit from. You want to be able to *see and feel the movement from where you are to where you want to be*.

These are the workhorse goals, the ones that really carry us from now to the end goal, and they deserve to be celebrated. Milestones is the perfect word for medium goals: they're telling you that you're making progress on your journey and show you how far you have left to go!

Small goals really are just that: things you can do anywhere between 'by the end of the day' and 'by the end of the week.' These are the things you need to be doing every day, better habits and good decisions—the fundamental unit of high-quality lifestyle change.

These are simple things like, "I'm bad at push-ups so today I'm going to work on them more closely." This is the penny in the jar that, after months, adds up to something worthwhile—they're the tiny choices that make 1% differences day by day and, without notice, produce amazing results.

You need to focus on these whenever possible, since they offer a kind of on-the-ground change that makes everything else possible!

PROCESSES ARE MORE IMPORTANT THAN GOALS

One of the focuses we need to lean into is prioritizing processes over goals whenever we can. Goals can be failed or achieved, but processes don't really care. They're also what you're going to spend most of your time dealing with, so they should be the bit you focus on most.

Processes include things like regular training, how you diet, how you prepare food, how you cook, what you do with your environment, and similar factors. These are processes because they're things you do repeatedly over time, and which produce a long-term trajectory of what you did and the results you got from it.

Focusing on processes is great because they determine the *trajectory* of your results, which is crucial because trajectory over time determines where you end up. When you look at timeframes like the rest of your life, the difference 1% can make in terms of your trajectory is **enormous**, so you need to zone in on these processes.

For example, nobody cares how motivated and intense you are in the gym if you're only turning up once a week or training at home every so often. Rather, a good process is being consistent and persistent, showing up regularly, doing the things you know you have to do, and going home for good food and rest.

The more we can shift away from goals and toward everyday behaviors, habits, and choices, the better we're able to change behavior and start improving who we are and how we act. This is why our everyday goals are important, and it's how we manage to achieve the medium goals—they are the result of repeated positive choices and habits.

It's totally reasonable to ask yourself how far you are from your goal, but it's always going to be **more** relevant to ask, "how am I moving toward that goal *today*?" This is what processes are all about, and it's why you need to prioritize consistent improvement over chasing a specific goal—the goal will come and go as you work on your process.

So will the one after that, and the one after that, and so on. That's because the keys to success in strength training are twofold, but also very simple.

CONSISTENCY AND PERSISTENCE

These are the two tools that are most important in fitness at any age (over 40s inclusive) and if you overlook them, your strength training journey won't progress the way you want it to. This is because consistency and persistence—always doing the right thing and sticking with it over time—are what separates you from your goals.

Imagine what you could do with your goals if you had 10 years of just doing the bare minimum. That's a lot more than you're getting right now—even those results, which aren't nearly maximal, are enormous.

This is why consistency is going to be key: doing something 80% correct, for example, over a year is more effective than 100% perfection for 6 months. This consistent, sustainable approach is what we're looking for: you don't need to live like an elite athlete, you just need to live better than you have been doing for a long time.

Time is the winning factor in your training, and all it takes is making good choices, regularly. **You cannot possibly fail your goal if you stick with it—the only thing that changes is the timing**. Better, stricter habits get you there quicker, but even the minimum viable effort will get you there *eventually*.

Focus on a system of exercise, diet, and lifestyle that you can maintain forever, and you can improve along the way, rather than insisting on things being perfect (and unsustainable) from the start.

SYSTEMS OVER MOTIVATION—BUILT TO LAST

The idea of motivation is a fickle one. This is tied closely to how you set your goals and expectations, and we want to rely on it as little as possible for training as well as for nutrition.

The idea is to make things systematic and obligatory, rather than relying on a burst of enthusiasm for them. The feeling of wanting to lose weight *will* come and go, depending on the tempting foods and tired mornings when you need to make good choices. Treating these habits like they're non-optional is always better.

You also want to set up systems and environments that make them easy. Have your gym bag packed in your car at all times, set out your workout clothes the night before, and (heaven forbid) get a good sleep so you're fresh when it counts most.

The idea is to give future you all the advantages you can in order to avoid the problems that you know trip you up. This means setting out reliable, easy meals that are relatively healthy and you know you can motivate yourself to eat instead of take-out, or just *going* to the gym even if you're not feeling it. Get something done and you're likely to find your motivation along the way.

Remember: Your behaviors affect your feelings more than the other way around. Get the behaviors right repeatedly and you'll start feeling better once you take the first step.

*"It's never too late to **CHANGE** old habits."*

— FLORENCE GRIFFITH JOYNER

PART II
NUTRITION

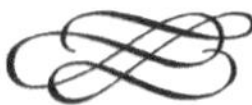

Nutrition is, in many ways, more important than exercise for most purposes. You could quite easily lose weight and get into better shape by changing your diet alone—it's roughly 80% of the process.

However, when it comes to eating to build muscle and gain strength, we need to be more active. You're going through a process of training to cause stress on the muscles, then fuel them for recovery and growth. Unlike regular 'dieting,' the idea here is to match up your hard work in training with an appropriate diet.

For this reason, we're going to look over the principles of nutrition and what you should focus on in order to get the most from good strength training exercises. These are simple things you practice and improve with over time; you don't need to get it all perfect right away, but each good habit you build on top of the last is a step in the direction of better results, and a better return on the time you put into your workouts.

FORGET EVERYTHING YOU THINK YOU KNOW

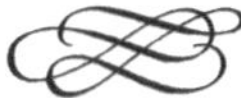

lmost everything you think you know about nutrition is either wrong or half-right, which is perhaps even more of a problem. The way we discuss nutrition in our culture is deeply flawed: we need to empty the cup in order to fill it up with clean water.

When was the last time someone told you that they were on a diet? Do you think they could have explained how and why that diet worked, if you asked them? Do you think it works at all?

The problem for most people when it comes to diets is that they actually don't understand how their body works. People are willing to work hard if they know the path to success, but the current stereotype of a diet involves cutting out anything enjoyable or filling and living on veggies and unseasoned chicken breast—or some overpriced dietary replacement drink.

The fundamentals of nutrition have never changed—humans have worked the same way for thousands of years, but you can't sell that because it's not sexy. However, getting these fundamentals correct is going to be the cornerstone of your success: you can't out-work a horrible diet.

THE NEW (OLD) FOCUS

We need to discard the new-age nonsense of cleanses and all-juice diets, without trying to be a bodybuilder living on bland and uninteresting foods for the sake of it. This is the approach of a scientific diet: find a balance between what you want and what science says is optimal.

You've got to prioritize the basics just enough to allow you to achieve your goals without making your diet unsustainable, leaving a little space for enjoyment of luxury foods in moderation. This helps keep everything balanced.

After all, you want you to be able to stick with this diet, and that's not possible when you drive the calories through the floor and have nothing enjoyable to eat.

THE PROBLEM WITH NUTRITION: SETTING UP MODERATION AND PROGRESSIVE IMPROVEMENT

The idea of how we tackle nutrition is simple: set up the basics of good dieting and then, from there, include moderate intake of luxury foods and continual substitutions for better foods over time.

This is the approach that produces results: get a ton of the work done with awareness and basics, then work on slowly tweaking it to get better and better with progressive, gradual improvements. You don't have to go from your normal diet to something perfect and flawless.

This reflects the kind of realistic expectations you want in your goals: start smaller, address the biggest issues, and then focus on specifics when these good habits are set up.

TRIAGE UNTIL THE BIGGEST PROBLEMS ARE SMALL PROBLEMS

What we do with diet is this: start by focusing on the biggest problems and priorities. Then, when that's done, we focus on the next biggest. You repeat this process until the biggest problem is actually really small and you've "accidentally" managed to remove 90% of the imperfections in a diet.

This is an approach that lets you work through at your own pace without dropping you in at the deep end or expecting you to change 50 things at once. Concentrate on one change at a time, make it stick, and then repeat the process again and again.

As I've mentioned above, clearly persistence and consistency are leading the way again. Now let's look at what the nutrition science says you need to focus on and how to deal with it—the **real** nutrition science!

BASICS OF NUTRITIONAL SCIENCE

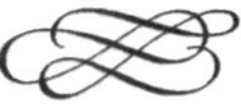

CALORIES

These are often demonized, but ***calories are just a measure of the energy that you get from eating and digesting a food***. This doesn't mean it's healthy or unhealthy—what's unhealthy is getting the wrong quantity of calories for your goal in a day or a week.

Calories only tell us what happens with weight, not what that weight is or what it does. Eating more calories than you use in a day means you're going to gain weight (as either muscle or fat), while eating less than you use in a day means you're going to lose weight (again, either as muscle or fat).

The amount you use in a day is an estimate called the Total Daily Energy Expenditure (TDEE), and we use this as our starting point for how much we need to eat in a day. You can log your food with mobile apps like MyFitnessPal to keep track of what you eat through a day.

This kind of tracking is awesome because, if nothing else, you'll come to understand what is in certain foods. This can be a huge part of the dietary process, showing you where you're over-eating, often without even knowing it!

People "on a diet" tend to restrict calories, as this is how you achieve fat loss, while muscle-gain diets are *usually* in a calorie surplus. Setting your own goals is key here to make sure you're getting the right quantity of calories.

You usually want to be around 300 to 500 calories above or below your TDEE. More than 500 under tends to be too restrictive and can cause more muscle loss, while more than 500 calories over the TDEE will likely cause more fat gain than intended.

These are also great lines for keeping progress sustainable and being able to commit to the process for an extended period of time. They also match up with the progress speed I mentioned above: 500 calories under your TDEE every day will produce around 1lb of fat loss per week, or around 0.5lb of muscle gain.

MACROS

Macronutrients are the major building blocks of food and are the most plentiful nutrients within it, hence the name. There are three macronutrients that each have an important role in the diet:

Proteins are one of the building blocks of cells and are primarily used in the body to repair or build crucial tissues, with muscle being one of those. Bones, tendons, muscles, and organs are all heavily dependent on proteins—more of them in the diet means better metabolism, better muscle growth, and prioritizing fat-burning when we eat under our TDEE.

Carbohydrates are the main short- and mid-term energy source for the body. They include sugars and starches, as well as the non-digestible *fiber,* which is key for metabolic and digestive health. Carbs are going to make up a decent portion of the diet and what matters is the quality of source you choose. Ideally, this means more starches and fiber, especially from pulses and whole grains.

Fats are important for cell membranes, keeping the brain healthy (especially as you age), and help with hormonal health. They're more calorie-dense than either protein or carbs, so you want to get less of them. They're also long-term energy sources, for when you run out of carbohydrates in the body.

MICROS

Micronutrients are vitamins and minerals—they're not any less important, they just don't tend to have calorie values. Your body doesn't use them for energy or as the building blocks of tissues, but they do play secondary and supporting roles to these processes, and you're going to run into major health risks if you're deficient in vitamins and minerals.

It's easy to look at it in an oversimplified way: micronutrients are all about health. They relate to things like performance results, but they're mostly important for keeping your organs healthy and functioning as intended.

There are 25 essential vitamins and minerals that you need to focus on, but they're all provided through a combination of lean proteins, choosing the right carb sources (like pulses and whole grains), and then a good quantity and variety of fruits and veg.

There are 12 essential vitamins:

- A
- B1
- B2
- B3
- B6
- B7
- B9

- B12
- C
- D
- E
- K

And 13 essential minerals:

- Iron
- Calcium
- Sodium
- Potassium
- Magnesium
- Zinc
- Iron
- Copper
- Manganese
- Phosphorus
- Chromium
- Iodine

These are a lot to remember, but just note that they're the ones to focus on. What we want to do is **avoid deficiency**, which is primarily done by eating the kind of diet outlined above, but also through the variety and range of plant foods in the diet.

Focus should go specifically to getting lots of B vitamins, vitamin D, and minerals like magnesium, potassium, and iron.

It's definitely worth getting your vitamin and mineral levels checked with your doctor whenever possible so you can look at what specifically is missing from your diet.

FOOD QUALITY

As we get through the basics, you can start looking at your sources of carbs and vitamins and minerals. Some sources are better than others for their concentration of pseudo-vitamins, but more specifically we're looking to focus on whole foods.

These are the kinds of "real foods" we want in the diet because they tend to contain fiber, better ratios of proteins to fats, and they're usually more nutrient dense. What you want to avoid is demonizing non-whole foods, though.

Some foods are specifically designed to get the best of a whole food, or are refined in ways that simply make them better to eat without compromising the nutritional or health qualities of the food. The idea is to get whole foods in the diet wherever possible and avoid **depending** on non-whole foods.

This is a good thing to work on in the long run, but it should not be your focus until you've already gotten your calories and macronutrients in place. Many people fail their diets by rushing straight to this step and ignoring the **more important stuff above!**

FOOD TIMING

You can get a little more benefit out of your food if you eat it at specific times. This is a step beyond food selection and it's where you really start getting into the fine details. It's not something you need to worry about too much, but here's a quick overview.

Carbs are better consumed closer to exercise, and consumed less further away from exercise and activity. Sugars, specifically, are best consumed very near exercise or even *during* in order to keep your energy levels up and maintain glucose levels during exercise. This has been related to improved performance and is the best time to get in that sugary snack you're in love with.

Proteins are best dosed regularly through the day if possible, but specifically after exercise and activity. Post-workout meals should focus on proteins and carbohydrates, as these are the resources that exercise depletes and eating them supports the systems that repair and develop muscles and tendons.

Fats should be consumed even further out of exercise than carbohydrates since they're a slower source of energy and can often sit heavily. We want to reduce, but not eliminate fat intake around the time of exercise to keep the digestive system happy, saving fats for breakfasts and evening meals after our workouts.

SUPPLEMENTS

You don't *need* supplements, but they can provide a great helping hand for a diet – whatever level you're at. Even if you're mastering the diet and putting 100% effort in, you can benefit from strategic supplement use.

We see this in elite athletes: people whose diets are perfect, but they're still using **multivitamins**, **protein** supplements, **creatine**, and **cod liver oil**, as well as an **effervescent**. These are the kinds of supplements you should look at.

Supplements allow you to top up your diet with compounds important for performance and health in a convenient way. They're ways of improving your intake without having to eat a ridiculous amount of fish, beef, or eggs, for example.

This is when concentrated sources are great—but, again, you shouldn't use them to replace a shortcoming in your diet. The idea is that they are *supplementary*: they're added on top of a good and developing diet, but they're not a replacement for good dietary habits.

A diet isn't just a collection of scientific principles about metabolism and nutrients. It's a habit change that has a person at the middle of it – and these factors need to be considered because they're going to be about your **experience** on a diet.

After all, science doesn't do the work for you: simply knowing what you need to do doesn't make it happen. That comes from the hard work of being self-aware with your diet and working on the bits that you're bad at, improving your habits day by day, and making good choices when that cake is calling to you.

Remember that dieting is a fallible process and you're going to make mistakes—you're going to stumble, and you're going to have bad days. The ideal response is to **just forget about it.** You want to avoid anything like guilt or a spiral of "I've failed, may as well give up" that you see so often.

*"No matter how many mistakes you make or how slow you progress, you are still **WAY AHEAD** of everyone who isn't trying."*

— TONY ROBBINS

PART III
TRAINING EXERCISES

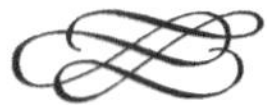

The exercises we use in this program are quite varied and will cover, between them, every muscle group in the body. I want to outline **why** they're chosen as they are, and hopefully offer you some personal education on which exercises are going to matter most, why, and provide a way of selecting exercises for yourself in future.

This section is going to cover the **what** and **why** of training exercises—from the warm-up to the workout—and why I think each of them deserves a spot in this program.

This part will also set the stage for the program itself—when you come to the program, you'll be familiar with all the exercises that are included and why you should be prioritizing them.

PRINCIPLES OF GOOD EXERCISE SELECTION

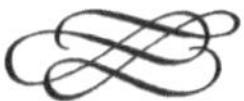

I could just tell you what exercise you should be doing, but that would be missing the point. What matters is choosing good exercises and understanding **why** they're the right exercises—you need to learn what has made them useful. why they're effective, and how they're selected.

Remember: getting your fitness together is as much of a process of self-education as it is just doing workouts and eating healthily. Understanding the what, why, and how of your strength training exercises is as important as understanding what role proteins play in the diet or which workout you're doing today.

I want you to be able to leave this section with a basic understanding of how you'd choose any exercise, or at least pick from a group of alternatives. That way, you've got a little more freedom and a lifelong skill, which are key to long-term improvement!

SCALING: REGRESSION AND PROGRESSION OPTIONS

One thing you want to look for is how easily an exercise scales up or down to meet your personal experience, strength, and skill levels. This is something we see with a lot of the best exercises that offer a good "on-ramp" to get to them.

These are important because we all come to exercise from a different medical and psychological background, so we want something that anyone can start with. This might mean changing the exercise to suit reduced experience, but that's fine because that is simply the fastest way of progressing for that person or situation.

There are many good examples of this—we can look at a simple movement like the lunge as an outstanding example. You can scale a lunge all the way back to a low step-up, then work through reverse lunges which are a little more challenging, then walking lunges, side lunges, and ultimately the Bulgarian split squat.

This is great because you can get on the path to progress at whatever level you're at, while also knowing that the strength, muscle, injury-resilience, and skill development results are going to be consistent well into the future. It regresses well, and it progresses well.

This is often true of larger compound exercises, such as the overhead press and the squat, and the simpler we get, the more room for scaling there tends to be. This does require learning a little bit about an exercise, but fortunately we're going to offer scaled options in our workouts in this book.

SKILL DEVELOPMENT

The more opportunities an exercise offers for practicing important skills, the better. To return to the lunge example, we're getting balance, single-leg strengthening, asymmetrical hip strength, some core work, and learning to support weight during movement.

These are skills we want to develop for life, but also for progressing through our exercises and getting better at movement. These are the keys to long-term control and stability benefits—and why are we exercising if not to move better?

Exercises that build key skills like this should be given some priority, and we always want to understand how an exercise carries over to other exercises and activities. This is especially true if you're new to exercise, since these skills are going to be under-developed.

MULTI-BENEFIT MOVEMENTS

This is closely related to the skill development section, but notably different.

This refers to the different kinds of structural effects that an exercise might have, as well as the role it plays in the workout plan. Does it combine two muscle groups we want to train? Does it build strength **and** power?

This kind of multi-benefit movement allows us to achieve a lot of results with a relatively smaller input of effort and skill-demand. It's a great thing to work on and—of course—the lunge is a great example.

It's a leg and hip movement, builds core strength, has tons of interesting variations, and helps us to improve mobility and balance alongside muscle and strength. I'm going to pack the workout program with this kind of exercise because the results are great, and your time is valuable.

ADAPTATION SPECIFICITY: STRENGTH, POWER, ENDURANCE, HYPERTROPHY

When you're choosing your own exercises, it's going to be important to make them specific to your goals. This applies at a number of levels, however.

First, it's about the adaptation you want: you're not going to get muscular with running, and you're not going to improve your 5k by bench pressing. The things we do produce more progress in *similar* activities, and less in *dissimilar* ones.

Equally, exercises can be more or less appropriate when compared with each other for certain goals. A jump will build leg power, while a squat will build leg strength (which is the basis of power, but not the same thing).

So, when it comes to exercise selection, you need to figure out your main goals and make sure your exercise choices are suited to that goal. Focus at least **near** the specific thing you're trying to improve.

CONVENTION: BASICS ARE GOOD, BUT THERE'S MORE TO LIFE

Exercise selection is often about justifying everything you do to align with one of your goals or something you're trying to achieve within a session, week, or training program.

Convention does tend to lead the way in some choices because it's good for the categories I've set out above: squats, lunges, presses, hip hinge movements, and rowing/pulling all have their classic entries.

We've all seen a bench press or a bicep curl, and these are clichés because they're good ways of achieving the result: a stronger chest or bigger arms. Equally, push-ups and sit-ups are popular forms of bodyweight exercise because they're easy and accessible.

Convention can be a good place to *start*, but it should also be met with the same question from above: *why* am I doing this? You can use convention to find inspiration, but it still needs to be vetted for appropriateness for your training experience and your goals.

You can also venture out beyond the conventional if you're willing to be even more skeptical. Novelty and variety can be a good driving force for progress: trying something new that you like the look of is fine, as long as you're not replacing everything in your workout plan all the time.

Focus on the basics, but allow yourself the freedom to experiment with your non-essentials—the stuff that's just about building some muscle and isn't very skill-intensive!

OUR FAVOURITE MOBILITY AND WARMUP EXERCISES

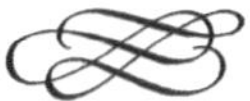

PRINCIPLES OF PICKING WARM-UP EXERCISES

We want to pick warm-up exercises that have a few key factors. Number one, they should have the scope for movement, since this helps to improve warm-up efficiency while also being effective in building better mobility and flexibility.

Additionally, exercises that can be scaled up or down are great, because then you can tailor your warm-up to your personal needs. This is key to making sure that you're getting the most from your time, and that you're not getting injured by over-exerting yourself in the warm-up.

I've put together a few of my favorites, where you should see what I mean by this, and how you can adjust them to your personal needs.

We also want to use exercises that are able to develop comfort and mobility in multiple joints at once. This is an awesome way of improving the quality of your warm-up time, and making sure that you're getting all your joints prepared for exercise.

Finally, we want to focus on exercises that are going to have at least some similarity to what we're doing within our workout. This is going to be important because *warm-ups are a chance to practice movement!*

If you can get moving better during your warm-ups, then you can improve your exercise technique for better muscle growth, better performance, and reduced injury risk. This is an all-round win that deserves the time and effort.

HIPS

Kneeling lunge

A key exercise for opening up the hips—make sure to keep your core and glutes active. You can improve this by moving backwards and forwards through the position to improve the effectiveness and make it more applicable to exercises like lunges and squats.

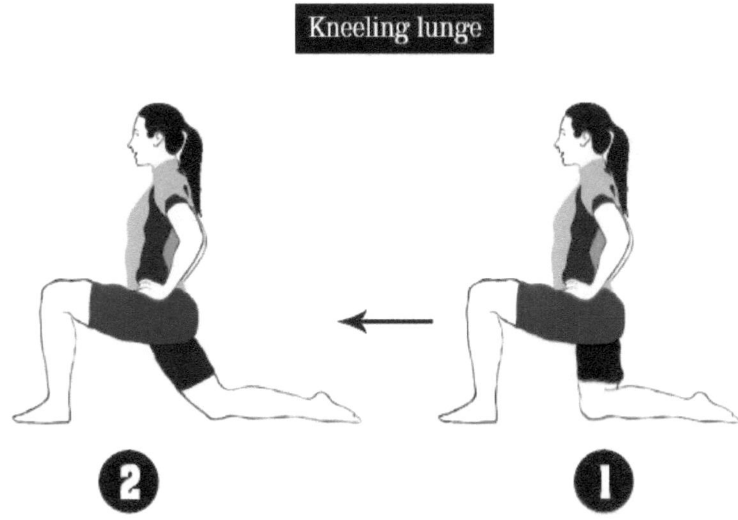

Glute bridge

A great way to get your glutes firing, which is key to getting stronger and keeping your lower back healthy. Squeeze and hold at the top, and you'll soon be feeling like your hips are more mobile at the front and more powerful at the back!

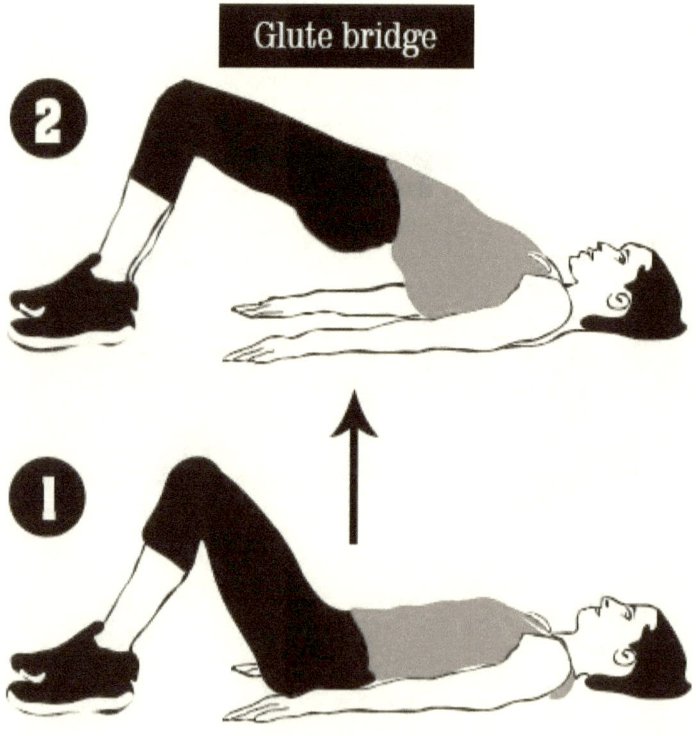

Pigeon stretch

This is an excellent glute stretch, though it can be a little challenging at first so take your time. We often neglect glute stretching, so regularly performing the pigeon is going to keep your hips healthy and avoid knee injuries.

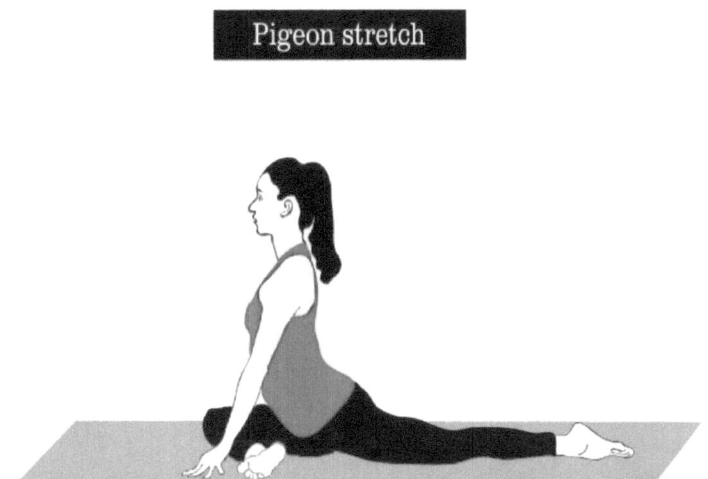

Partial cossack squat

Cossack squats are awesome for opening up the hips, getting the knees and ankles prepared for exercise, and waking up the core. They can be challenging, so be prepared to start with *partial* movements and focus on control and balance as you go.

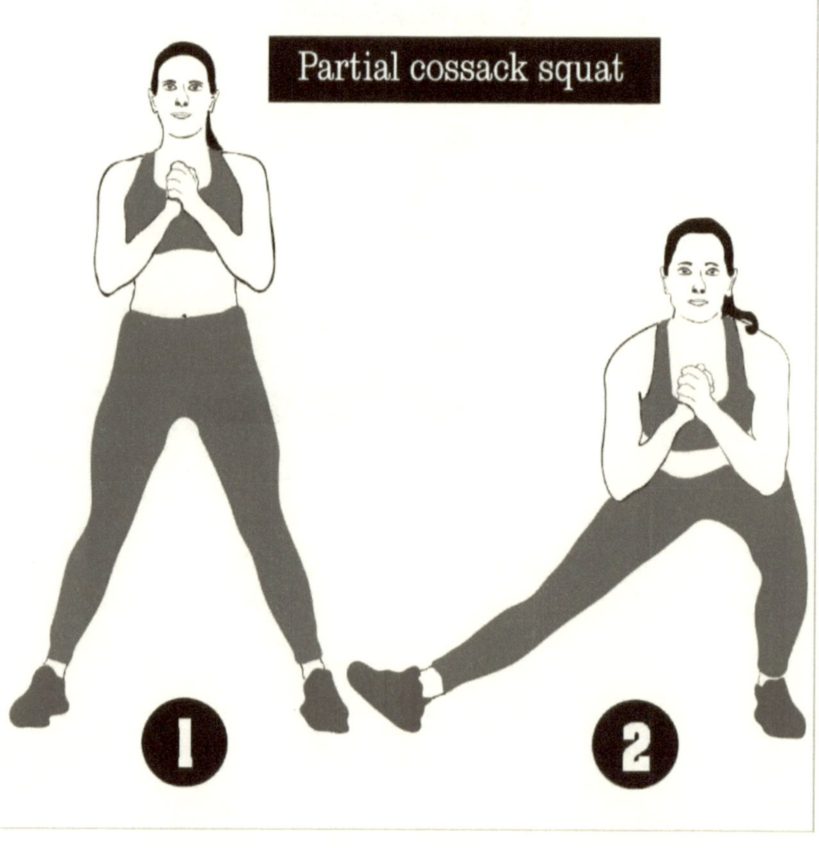

Hinge drill/Good morning

Developing a good hip hinging pattern isn't optional—you need to learn how to move your hips while keeping your back in one place. The broomstick hip hinge drill is perfect for this. You can really wake up your hamstrings and get them feeling looser with this movement.

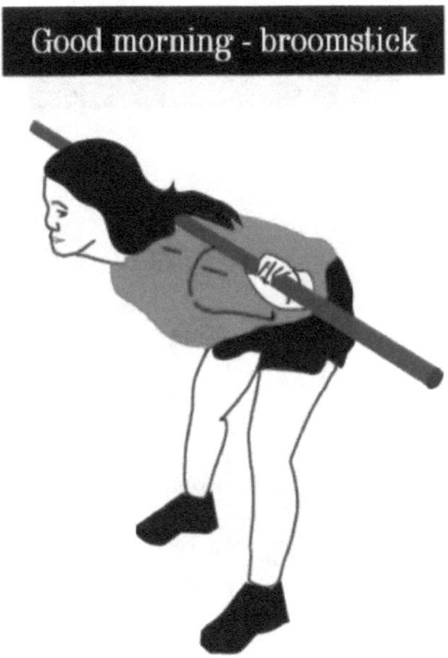

Straddle stretch

This is a great starting point for many really effective stretches. Equally, it's a great way of getting your hips open and stretching out the lower back, inner thighs, and hamstrings.

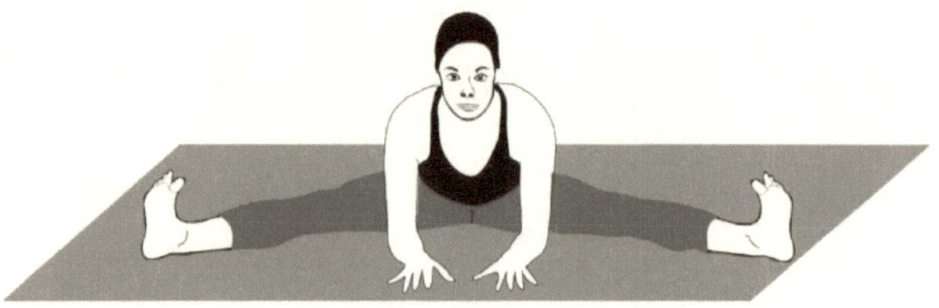

SHOULDERS

Dislocates

This is simple: work your shoulders through their full range of motion. Get comfortable with all of it! Think about keeping the stick/band as far away from your body as possible at all times, and never be passive.

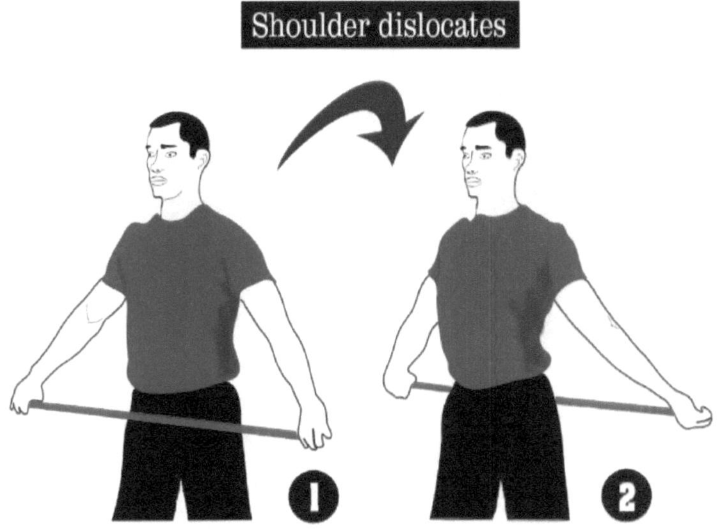

Pull-aparts

These are ideal for opening up the chest and getting the upper back involved in the motion of your shoulder. This is crucial for proper movement and many people will benefit from it in terms of posture, as well as strength and mobility.

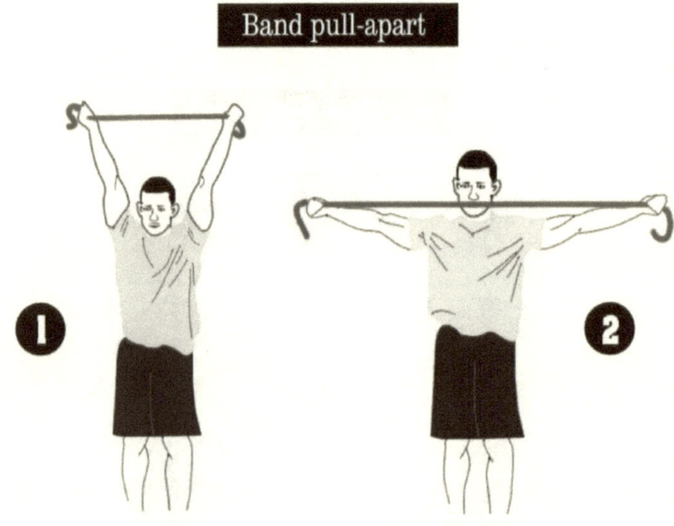

Chest stretch

This is a classic stretch, helping to loosen off the often-tight chest muscles that roll the shoulders forward. Again, a great postural exercise—and one you should vary between shoulder-height and higher variations, making sure to open up all the muscles in the chest.

Preacher and offset preacher stretch

Preacher stretches are perfect for opening up the lats, as well as getting your shoulders moving in multiple directions. Use a combination of normal and side/offset versions of the stretch to make sure you're getting a complete warm-up for the upper back.

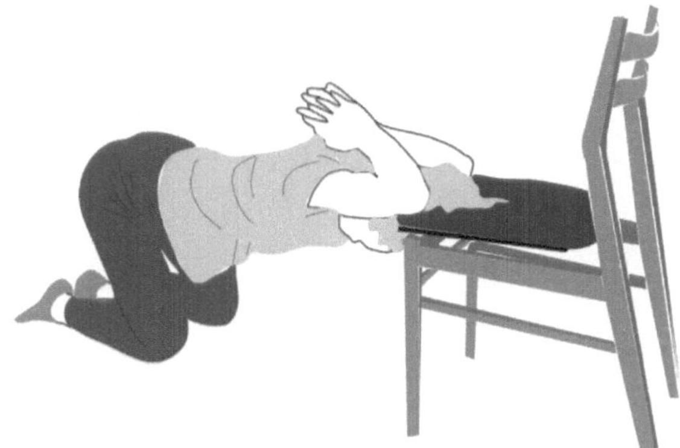

Underhand stretch (mild)

The seated shoulder stretch can be quite challenging because most of us have neglected shoulder extension, so now we're all tight. It's an excellent way of stretching the shoulders and even the neck/trap muscles, if you're patient and consistent with it.

SPINAL WARM-UP

Dead-bugs and bird-dogs

These are two great exercises for preparing your spine for exercise. They build core strength, teach you how to balance your rotation in the spine, and will naturally keep the spine healthy and stable during exercise. Pause in the end positions for both exercises, focusing on keeping the core in one place throughout the movements.

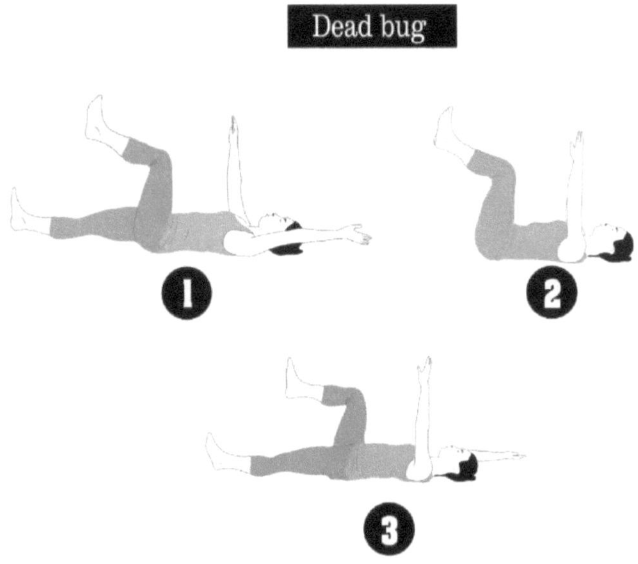

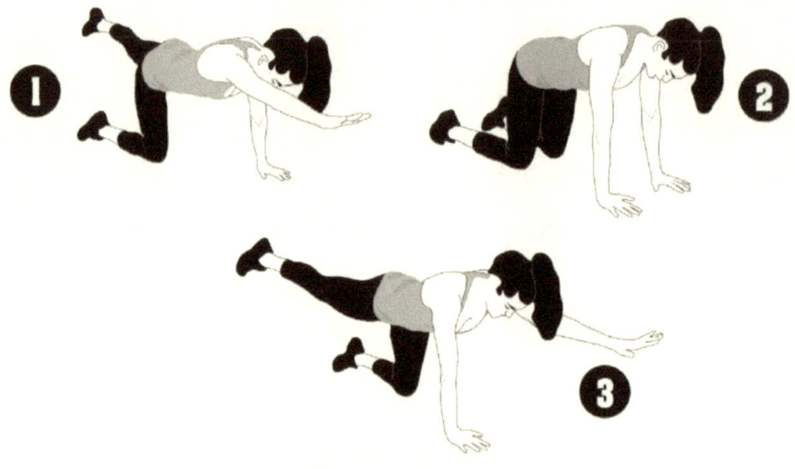

Bird dog
1
2
3

Plank variations

Planks are perfect for getting your core ready for exercise. They'll help reinforce proper hip-spine position and engage your abdominal muscles. Get a few 20-second holds on the normal plank and the side plank to really wake everything up and make sure you're taking care of your core.

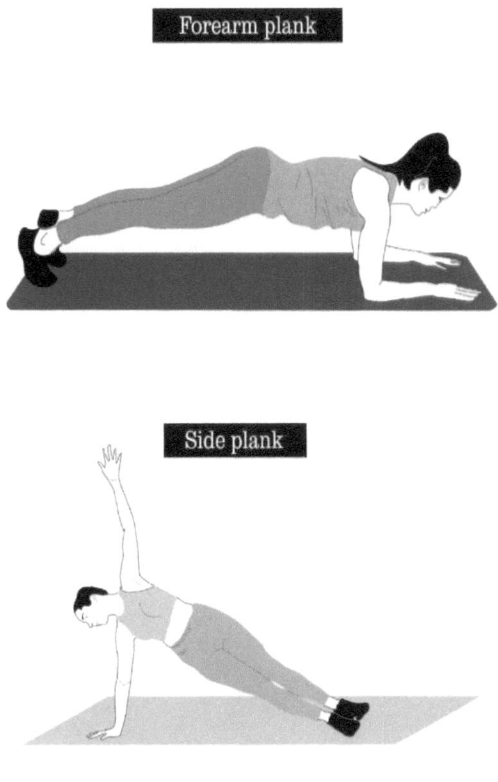

LEGS

Single leg quad stretch

This kneeling quad stretch is a great way of opening up the hip flexor and reducing strain on the knee itself. It can be developed patiently and even performed with both legs as you get stronger, more mobile, and more confident with the stretch.

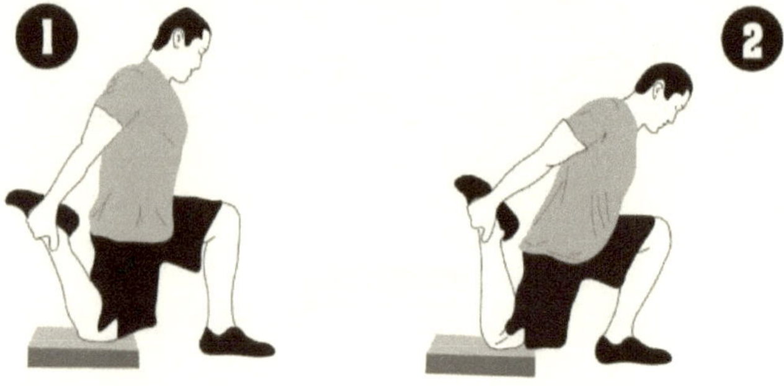

Standing/kneeling hamstring stretch

This is like the quad stretch mentioned above, but for the other side of the knee. It helps you to move the hamstring through full range—a muscle that gets *very* tight for most people due to lots of sitting, not much hip hinging, and weakness.

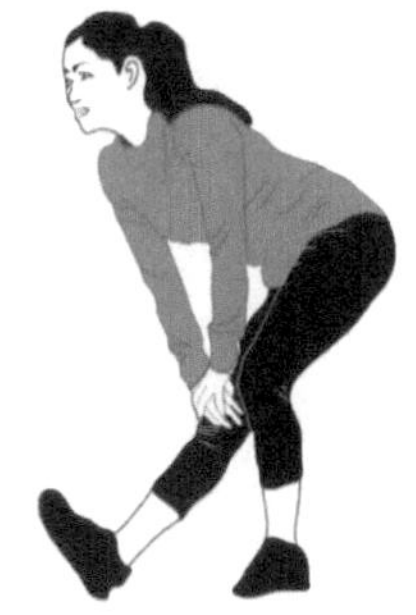

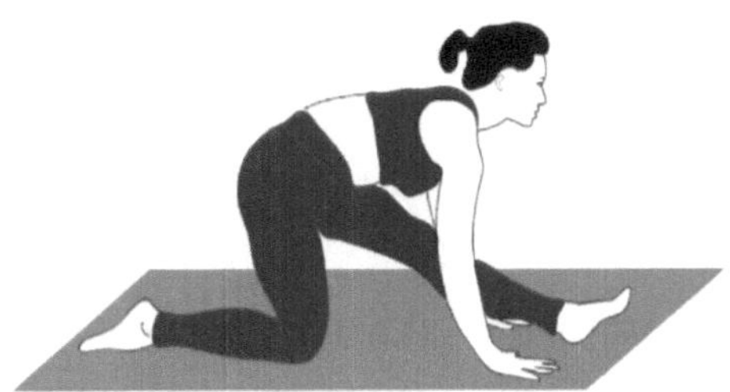

MOVEMENT PREP + PRACTICE

Once you've gone through these warm-up exercises, you need to perform light versions of your strength exercises for warm-ups. This is often, in the example of weight training, performing sets at 25%, 50%, 75%, and 90% of the intended workout weights.

This should also be performed with fewer reps as you increase weight, and jumps should always be smaller than those before to ensure you're not overexerting yourself during the warm-ups or taking unpredictable weight jumps.

Here's what a warm-up might look like for a set of 5 squats at 100kg:

- Empty barbell (20kg) for 5 reps
- 50% (50kg) for 5 reps
- 75% (75kg) for 3 reps
- 90% (90kg) for 2 reps

Again, the goal is to work on technical changes in movement and make sure everything looks and feels okay. This prepares the mind and body for the intensity and effort expected in the working sets.

PRELIMINARY FITNESS ASSESSMENT

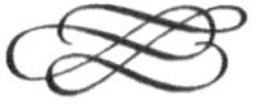

*B*efore starting to work out, you need to assess your physical condition, including muscular strength and endurance, overall flexibility, and cardiovascular endurance. This preliminary evaluation provides you with a baseline from which you can evaluate your own progress.

Before starting this assessment, discuss with your medical doctor any medical or health contraindications regarding specific exercises or positions. You may request a Graded Exercise Text (GXT) from your doctor to understand your oxygen consumption and intake, prior exercising; it is also called an exercise stress test. Your doctor will need to interpret the results for you. According to the American College of Sports Medicine (Balady 2000), such GXT is not required prior to starting vigorous exercise if you are an asymptomatic

40-year-old or younger male, or a 50-year-old or younger female.

EXERCISE INTENSITY AND OXYGEN INTAKE

A moderate exercise regimen will put you into an intensity of 40% to 60% of your maximum oxygen uptake capacity (VO2 max). A more vigorous one will bring you from 60% to 80% of such capacity. However, if you are new to working out and have lived a relatively sedentary lifestyle, you will want to target the moderate regimen first, to avoid overloading yourself too fast.

You also need to consider the exercise intensity, referring to how much energy is used when you are exercising. It is important that you do not train above the right intensity for you, as this may lead to no visible improvement or an overexertion of muscles, and perhaps even injury.

TARGET HEART RATE

The **target heart rate (THR)** is a good indicator of that, as it is best to maintain your heart rate within an age-based range to ensure good cardiovascular function. To assess the intensity of an exercise, try holding steady conversation. According to the ratings of perceived exertion (RPE), it should be difficult but not impossible (4-6). If you can talk easily (RPE 2-3), increase the intensity. This is according to the <u>revised Borg scale of RPE</u>.

To calculate your THR, estimate it by first identifying your maximum heart rate (<u>see Heart Website</u>). Subtract your age from 220 for men and 226 for women. For instance, a 55-year-old woman will have a Maximum Heart Rate of (226-55=)171 beats per minute. The THR range of 55%-60% advised here will be 94 bpm-102 bpm.

This means moderate-intensity physical activity for a 55-year-old will require that the heart rate remains between 94 and 102 bpm. More vigorous activity will lead to the THR to be between 60% and 75%, implying a THR for this 55-year-old woman of 102 to 128 bpm.

PRELIMINARY ASSESSMENT OF MUSCULAR STRENGTH

To assess muscular strength, it's important to have warmed up your muscles beforehand. One repetition only is needed, but one at the maximal resistance (1RM). For the upper body, a chest press of an Olympic bar is a good test; this should be done with someone next to you to help with the loading and unloading, and in case of failure. For the lower body, one repetition of maximum resistance of leg press is a good way to assess your legs' strength.

PRELIMINARY ASSESSMENT OF MUSCLES' FLEXIBILITY

To assess the flexibility of your muscles, there are several techniques. The zipper stretch measures the shoulders' flexibility. Place your right hand over your right shoulder and bring the left hand in the back. Try to connect them. If someone can take a picture of the position of your arms at the time, it will give you a starting point for your shoulder flexibility.

For the lower back and hamstrings, sit on the floor and extend your legs in front of you, with the knees as close to the floor as possible. Press your feet against a wall or a box and lean forward as far as possible without moving the knees. Assess how far down your legs your hands can touch.

PRELIMINARY ASSESSMENT OF MUSCULAR ENDURANCE

Squats, push-ups and sit ups are used to test your muscular endurance. Men should use the standard push-up, called military style, on hands and toes, while women can use the position with bent knees on the floor. The hands have to be on either side of the chest and the back straight.

For sit ups, lie on the floor with your knees bent upwards and your hands on your thighs. Contract your abdominal muscles and raise yourself high enough for your hands to touch your knees. Be careful not to pull at the neck and keep your lower back on the floor.

Squats are done with your feet flat on the ground, hip width apart. Exhale and get down in a seated position (maximum 90°). Don't lock your knees, as this could damage your joints. Do as many push-ups, sit ups, and squats as possible while keeping good form. These exercises leading to failure give you an idea of your muscular endurance.

If you suffer from chronic conditions, such as hypertension or diabetes, before you attempt the following workout plan, it is crucial that you prepare and fortify your cardio-respiratory system by training three times a week, at least. This is best done on a treadmill starting for 15 min, gradually increasing to 30 minutes.

STRENGTH TRAINING EXERCISES

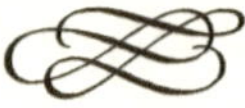

$\mathcal{A}$s lack of adequate muscular strength leads to decreased musculoskeletal functions in an aging population, strength training exercises are focused upon here. Strength is both the ability to contract muscles with a given force, as well as the ability to apply musculoskeletal force against an external object.

When training such exercises, it is crucial to maintain good posture. Having good posture in everyday situations as well as when working out is crucial, as it impacts the alignment of the bone joints and the muscles. Posture is the way the body holds itself when sitting, standing, lying down, or moving.

It is beneficial for everyone to practice exercises that benefit the posture. These tend to be exercises that favor balance and the symmetrical development of muscles. Weak erector spinae muscles of the lower back affect the ability to achieve and sustain an erect trunk when standing and walking. This is a problem that often affects older people. Back extension is a good exercise that targets these specific muscles.

COMPOUND EXERCISES AND ISOLATION EXERCISES

Compound exercises are crucial to many fitness programs. Unlike isolation exercises that are performed with weight machines, compound exercises focus on functional fitness developed by exercises that simulate real-life movements or activities.

Compound exercises are multi-joint movements that work several muscles or muscle groups at once. For instance, a squat engages the quadriceps, the glutes, the hamstrings, the calves, the lower back, and the core.

These exercises have the advantage of translating common movement patterns into workouts as well as working several muscles at once. These are beneficial as they maintain an elevated heart rate, offering additional cardiovascular benefits. As a consequence, they also burn more calories.

On the other hand, isolation exercises work only one muscle, muscle group or joint at a time, such as the biceps curl. All these can be performed on the machines found in gyms, or by using weights in a gym or at home. After an injury, it is not uncommon for a specialist to recommend the use of specific machines, as they enable good form while isolating the use of the targeted muscle group. By isolating a specific muscle, you activate it in a more precise manner, which may sometimes be necessary in order to increase its strength.

I recommend that you include both compound and isolation exercises in your workout routines. The compound exercises allow for a full body workout while the isolation exercises complement the program.

PROGRESSIVE OVERLOAD

This principle in weightlifting implies increasing the stress applied on the musculoskeletal system to continually gain in muscle size, strength, and endurance.

Through resistance training, your body adapts to the weight, meaning that it will gain strength, and your cardiovascular system will gain endurance. This is further developed in the strength month of the proposed workout.

As appropriate weights and resistances are unique to all individuals, no standards are given here. Instead, the formula enabling you to identify the right individual training method is explained.

WHAT DO YOU NEED TO TRAIN AT HOME?

In a gym, you will have most machines and free weights available. If you wish to train at home, you will need:

- **A yoga mat**. This should be thick enough that sitting on your tailbone won't be uncomfortable.
- **Resistance bands**. These vary in resistance and strength and can be used for stretching or to replace specific machines as they provide the required resistance. There are small ones (approximately 30 cm in diameter) and longer ones (approximately 1 m in diameter). The longer ones are more versatile and are referred to in our section on home workouts.
- **Dumbbells**. A range of dumbbells with weights that are manageable for you, as well as some that are challenging for you, is imperative. Dumbbells are preferred over barbells or kettlebells.

With this selected equipment, you will be able to train at home as well as in a gym.

EXPLANATIONS OF EXERCISES IN THE WORKOUT PLAN

All the exercises mentioned in the workout plan in the next chapter are listed here, divided into compound and isolation exercises.

The form of the following exercises has been detailed to enable you to perform them without relying on external sources or references.

ISOLATION EXERCISES

Standing calf raise

Target muscles: Calf (gastrocnemius)

1. While standing with your feet hip-width apart, press up on your toes, extending the sole of your feet. Pause at the top while your calves are fully contracted.

2. Release slowly and come back to the starting position.

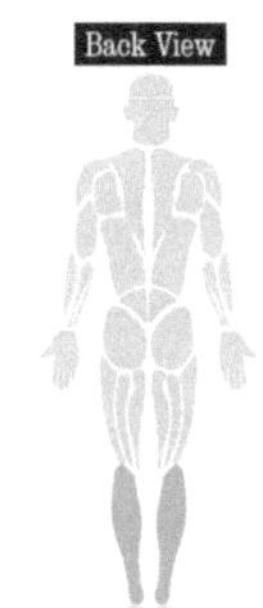

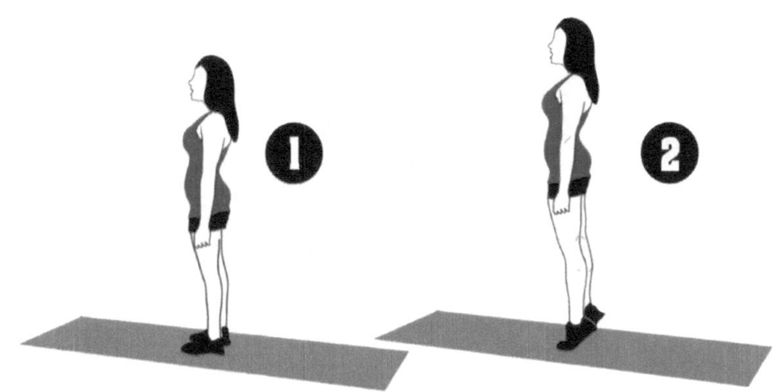

Seated calf raise

Target muscles: Calf (soleus)

1. Using the machine, sit with the knees firmly held by the roller.

2. Apply pressure to your toes and lower heels. You can add weight to the machine for added resistance.

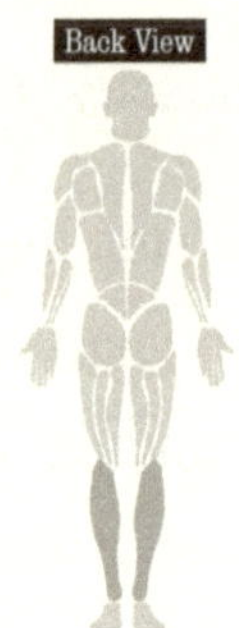

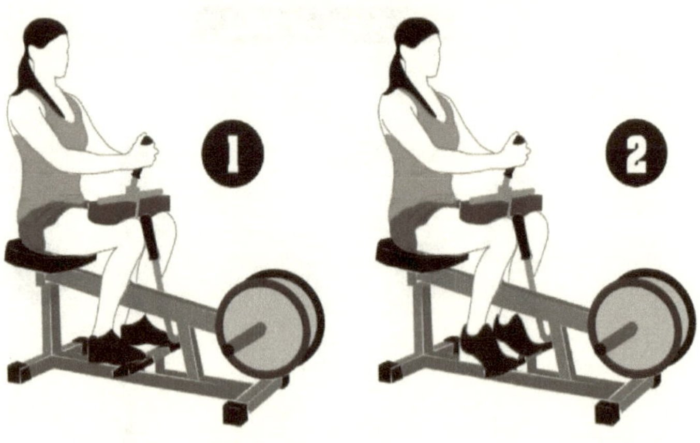

Without the machine, this can be replaced by standing calf raise.

Leg extension

Target muscles: Quadriceps

1. On a machine, extend your leg, avoiding full extension or locking the knee.

2. Adapt the resistance of the machine.

3. Hold the extension for 3 seconds.

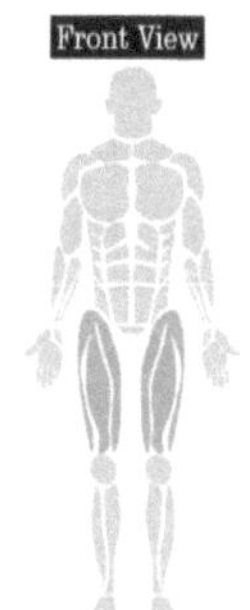

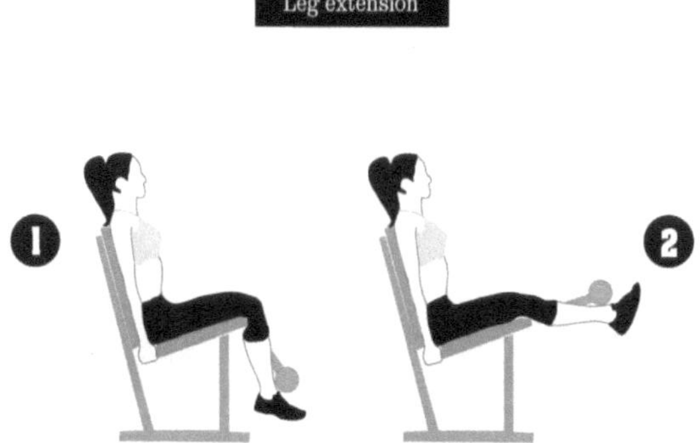

Home alternative:

Without a machine, you can do the same movement using a resistance band, securing it to your other leg or to an object.

Leg curl

Target muscles: Calf, hamstrings

1. On a machine, bend the knee toward the seat, contracting the hamstrings. Make sure the thighs and hips are firmly against the seat.

2. When you have reached the full range of motion, slowly raise the roller of the machine.

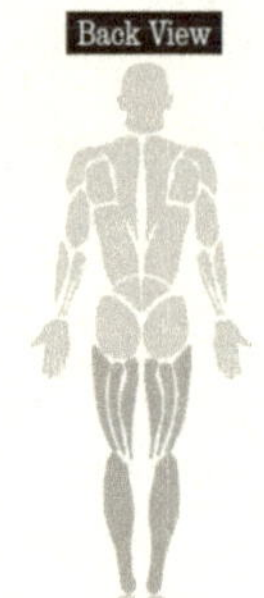

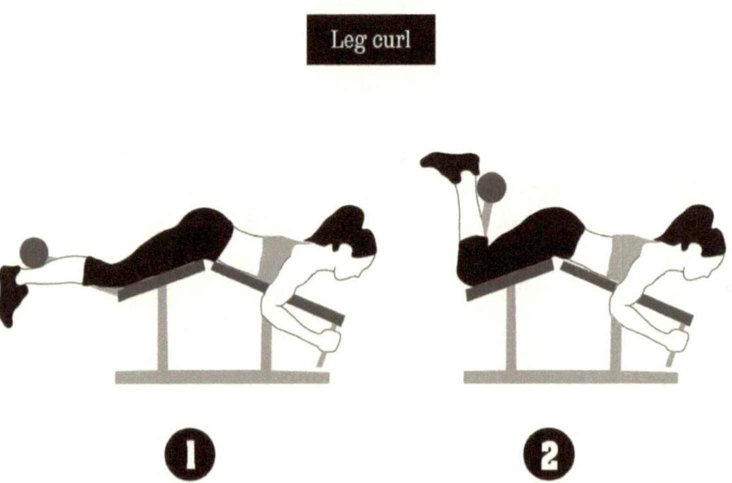

Home alternative:

1. Without a machine, lie prone and slowly bend the knee.
2. Place a resistance band at your feet, extending one leg while the other leg maintains the band.

Seated lateral raise

Target muscles: Lateral deltoid

1. In a seated position with your feet firmly grounded and your arms hanging down by your side, hold dumbbells in each hand with your palms facing each other. It is easier to sit at the end of a bench.

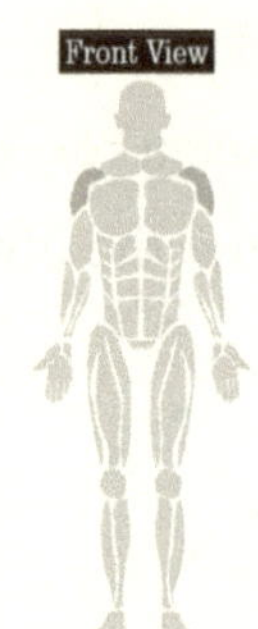

2. Raise your arms to the side, keeping your arms straight without locking the elbow. Pause at the top where your arms are parallel to the floor.

3. Inhale and bring your arms back down in a controlled manner.

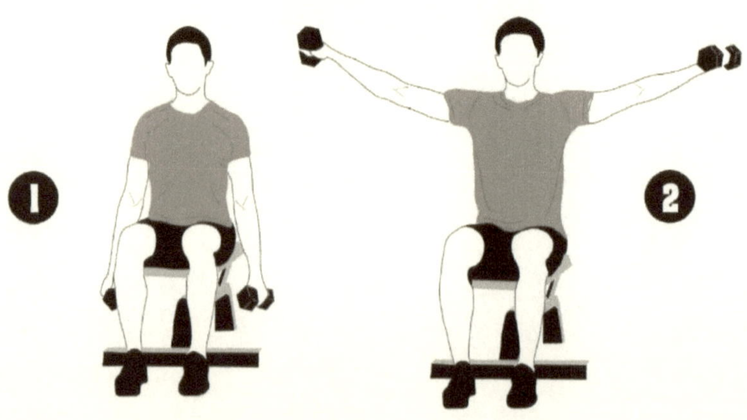

Standing lateral raise

Target muscles: Lateral deltoid

This exercise follows the same structure as the Seated lateral raise, but it works your stability during the workout.

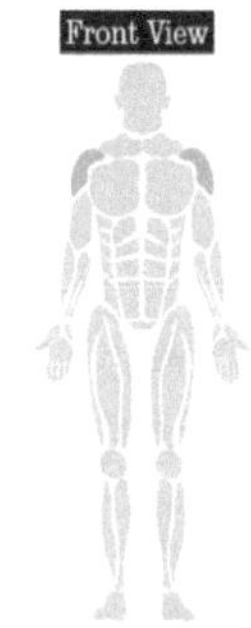

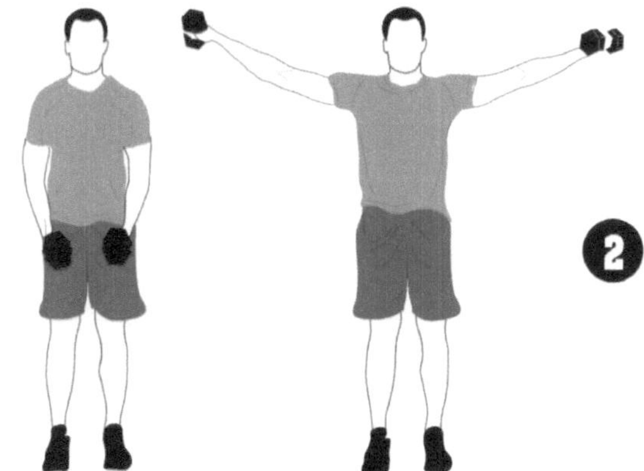

Biceps curl

Target muscles: Biceps

1. In a standing position, hold dumbbells in each hand. Your elbows should be on your sides and your forearms should extend in front of your body.

2. Bending your elbows, bring the dumbbells all the way up to your shoulder.

3. Hold the position while contracting the muscle and exhaling.

4. While inhaling, bring the weights down slowly.

You can also use barbell for this exercise.

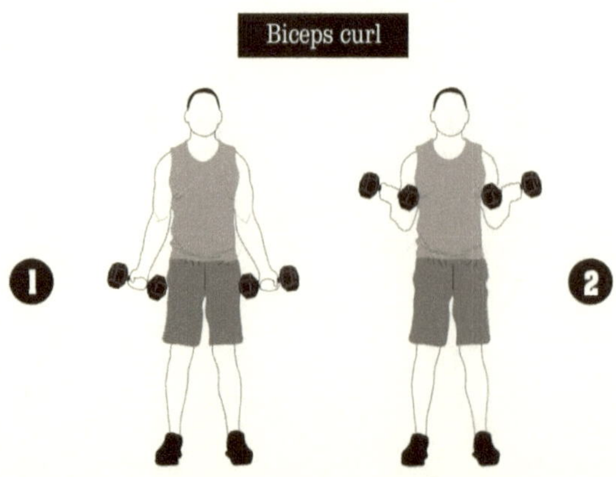

Single-arm isometric biceps curl

Target muscles: Biceps

1. Stand straight with your feet hip-width apart, holding dumb-bells in each hand with palms facing forward. Your elbows should be tucked and your fore-arms should extend slightly in front of your body.

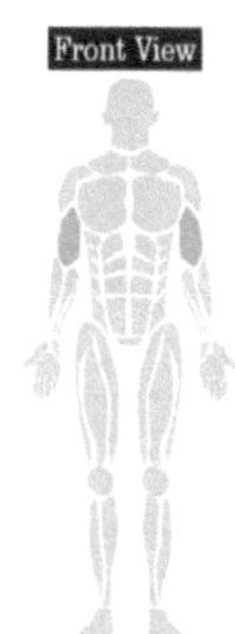

2. Bend your left elbow to about 90° and hold this position in an isometric fashion, maintaining a contraction in the muscle.

3. As you exhale, curl the weight in your right hand all the way up to your shoulder. Hold the position at the top.

4. While inhaling, bring the weight down in your right hand slowly back to the starting position. Do a few more reps with this arm.

5. Switch sides, and repeat the exercise with equal amount of reps.

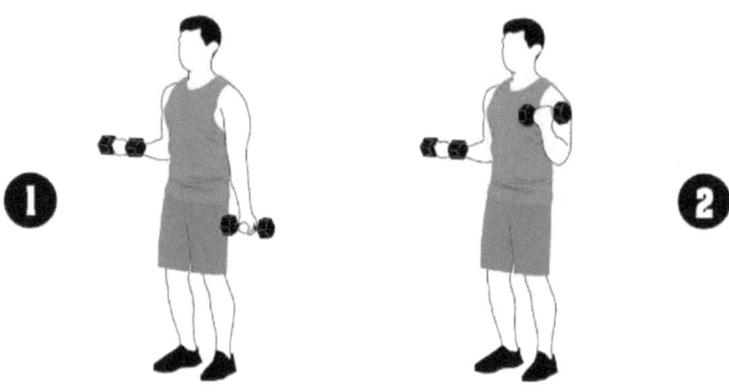
Single-arm isometric biceps curl

Bent-over reverse fly

Target muscles: Rear deltoid

1. Stand with your feet hip-width apart and knees slightly bent. Maintain a straight back and bend forward at the hips to about 90°.

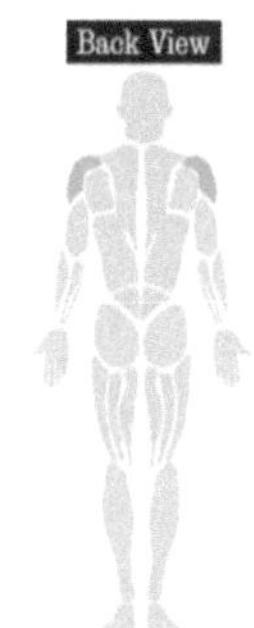

2. Holding the dumbbells with your elbows slightly bent and palms facing each other, raise your arms to the side until they are parallel to the floor before bringing them back down in a controlled form.

Back extension

Target muscles: Erector spinae

1. Place your thighs on the pads
of the machine.

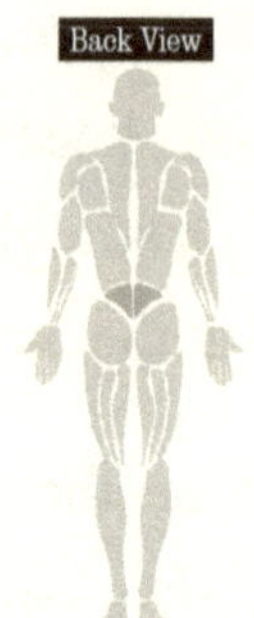

2. Secure your feet, and keep
your arms crossed in front of
your chest.

3. Begin with your torso and legs
aligned, take a deep breath in and
bend at the waist to lower your body towards the ground to
about 90°.

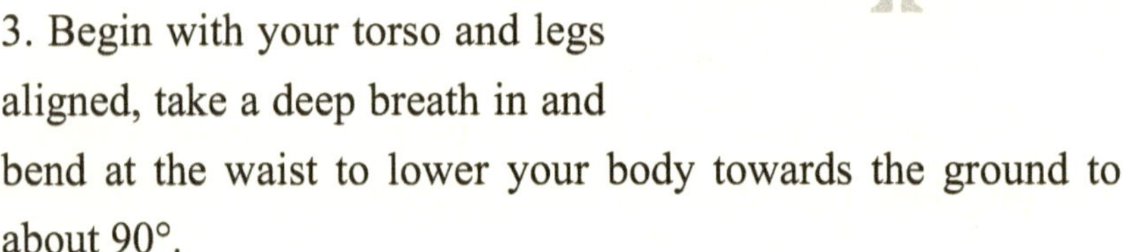

4. Engage your core.

5. Exhale and raise your torso back to the starting position.

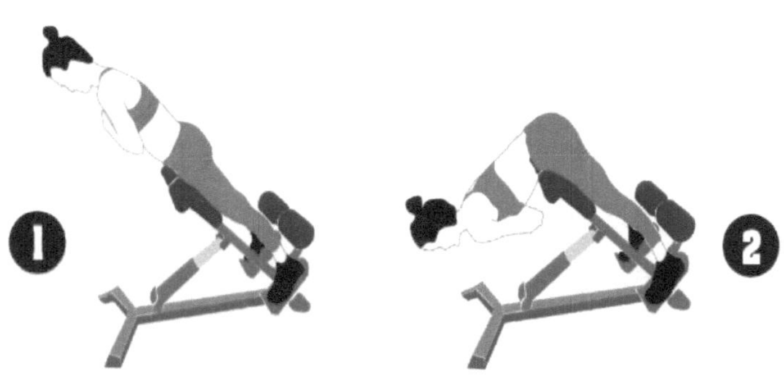

Home alternative:

This exercise can be done at home with someone holding your legs, or it can be replaced by the Superman exercise.

Overhand lat pulldown

Target muscles: Latissimus dorsi

1. Grab the bar of the machine with a wide overhand grip, keeping the torso upright.

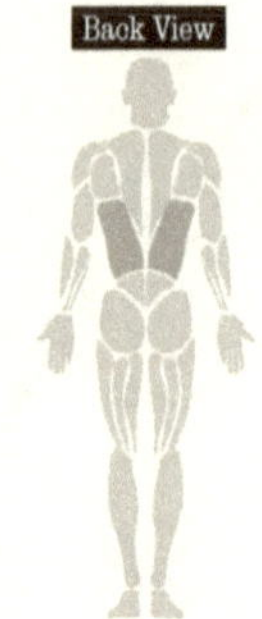

2. Retract the shoulder blades and pull the bar down towards your upper chest. Be careful not to make your grip too wide, as this involves other muscles.

3. Contract your latissimus dorsi at the bottom of the move-ment and exhale.

4. Hold this position before releasing the bar back up.

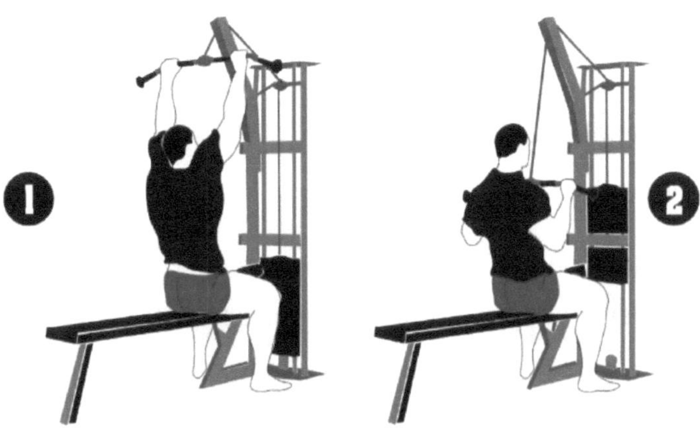

Home alternative:

Without a machine, you can do the lat pulldown with a loop resistance band. With your arms raised, place the loop band around your wrists and maintain a slight tension in the band. Pull the band apart, bringing the band behind your head and keeping your elbows bent. This makes you squeeze your shoulder blades and contract the latissimus dorsi muscle. Exhale at this point and return to the starting position with your hands overhead.

Supinated lat pulldown

Target muscles: Latissimus dorsi, biceps

1. Grab the bar of the machine with a wide underhand grip (palms facing you), keeping the torso upright.

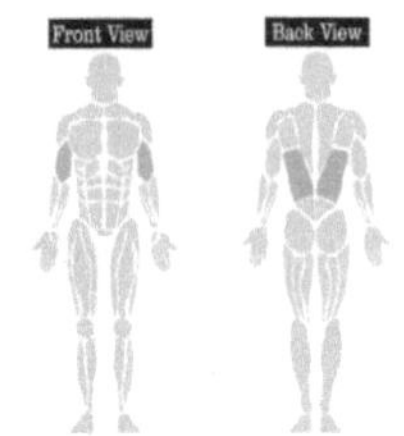

2. Retract the shoulder blades and pull the bar down toward your upper chest. Be careful not to make your grip too wide, as this involves other muscles.

3. Contract your latissimus dorsi at the bottom of the movement and exhale.

4. Hold the position before releasing the bar back up.

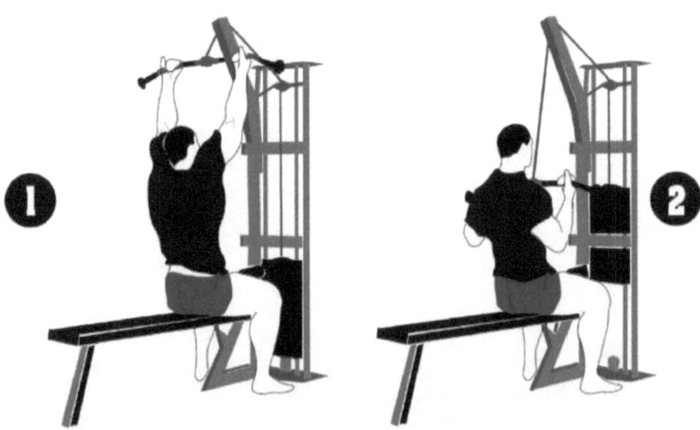

Machine chest press

Target muscles: Pectoralis major, deltoids, triceps

1. On the machine, press your back to the seat and push against the handles.

2. Hold the position in extension, then bring back the handles.

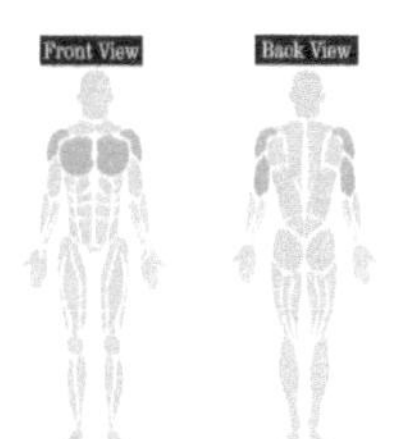

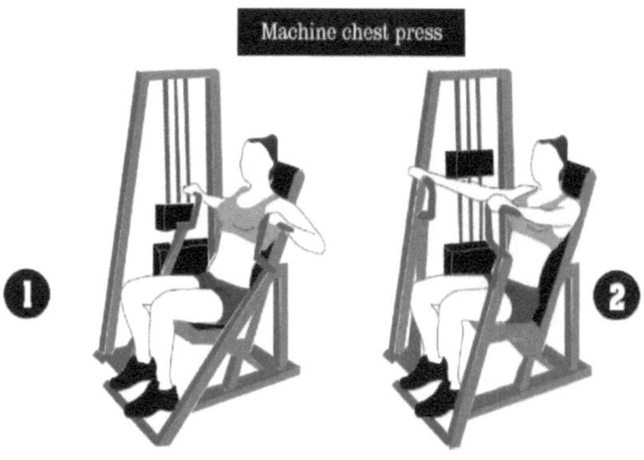

Home alternative:

This position can be done without a machine by placing a resistance band below your back with one end in each hand. This changes the dynamic of the movement, with the resistance being on a push motion, but it activates the same muscles as the machine equivalent.

Cable chest crossover

Target muscles: Pectoralis major

1. On a dual cable machine, set the pulleys at chest height.

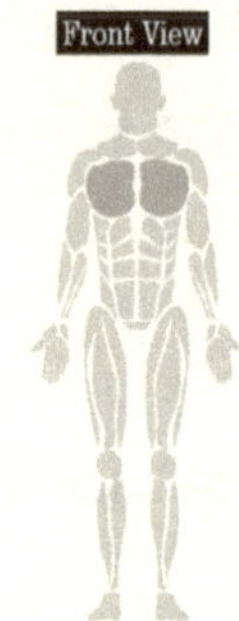

2. Standing between the two poles, grab the handles with your palms facing forward and take one step forward to create tension in the cable, keeping your back straight.

3. Stretch your arms out to your sides and maintain a slight bend in your elbows, keeping the shoulder blades retracted. This is the starting position.

4. Pull the cables forward and inward in an imaginary arc until your arms just cross each other in front of your body. Pause here and squeeze your chest.

5. Release the cables slowly back to the starting position. Switch the forward foot with each new set.

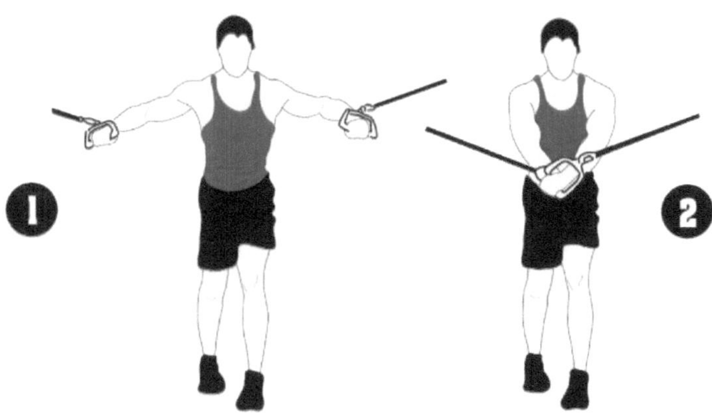

Home alternative:

This exercise can be done at home with a resistance band attached firmly behind the back to poles or any other rigid structure.

Triceps pushdown

Target muscles: Triceps

1. Using the cable machine, in a standing position, lean slightly forward with a straight back and knees slightly bent. Attempt to push down the rope and hold the position.

2. Exhale at this stage.

3. Inhale while flexing the elbows again.

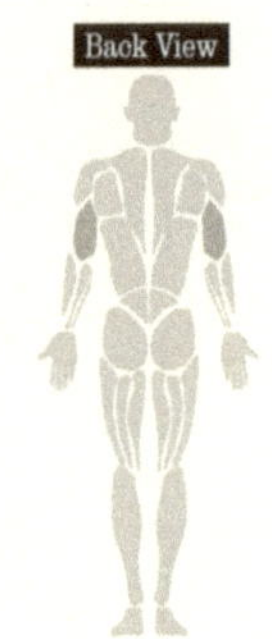

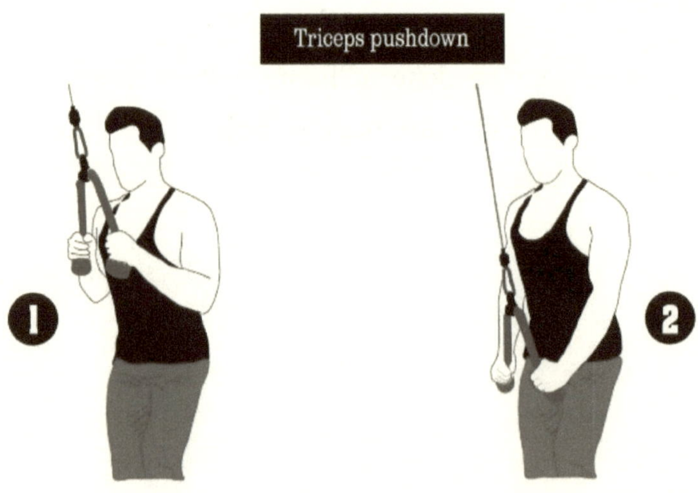

Home alternative:

Without a machine, a resistance band may be used when attached to the top of a door or another elevated solution. The movement is the same.

Supinated triceps pushdown

Target muscles: Triceps

1. Using the cable machine, in a standing position, lean slightly forward with a straight back and knees slightly bent. With your hands holding the straight bar in a supinated (underhand) grip, push down the bar and hold the position. This different grip changes the focus of the stress on the medial head of the muscle.

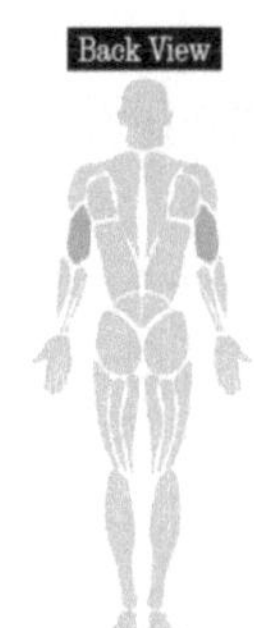

2. Exhale at this stage.

3. Inhale while flexing the elbows again.

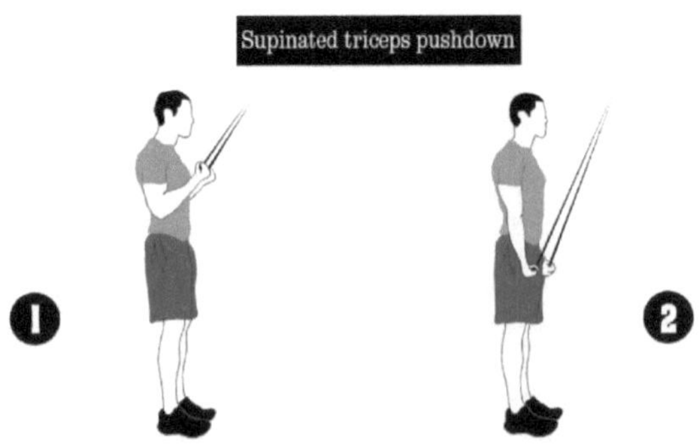

One-arm overhead triceps extension

Target muscles: Triceps

1. While standing, exhale as you lift the dumbbell with one arm until it is fully extended with palms facing the roof and elbows facing forward.

2. Slowly lower the dumbbell behind your head until you feel a good stretch in your triceps and return to the starting position.

3. Repeat with the other arm.

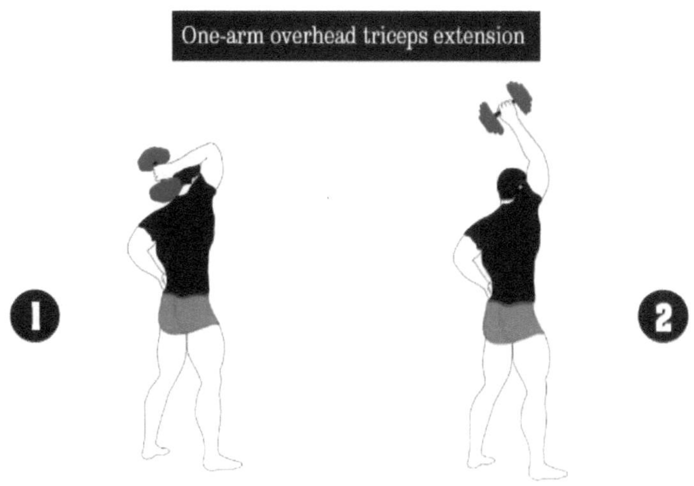

Face pull

Target muscles: Rear deltoid

1. Using the cable machine, reach up and grab the handles with your palms facing down.

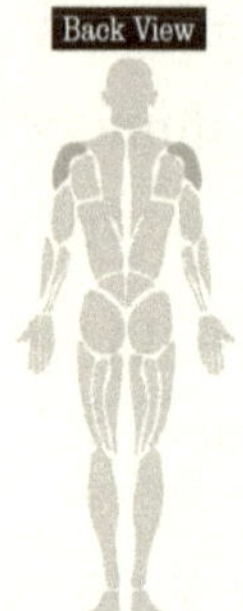

2. Step back until your arms are fully extended.

3. Engage your core and lean back slightly, at an approximate angle of 20°. Pull the rope toward you at face level and engage your shoulders.

4. Slowly release the resistance of the rope.

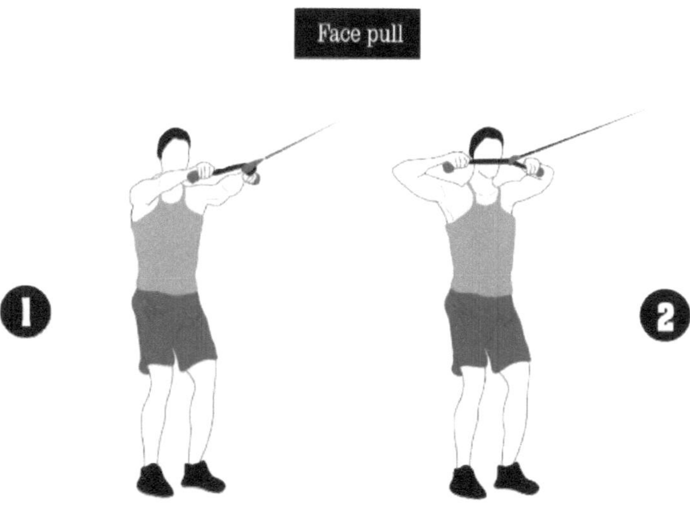

Home alternative:

This exercise can be done without a machine by hooking a resistance band to an elevated point, such as the top of a door or wardrobe.

<u>Static crunch</u>

Target muscles: Rectus abdominis

1. Lie supine, with your back and feet on the floor, keeping your knees bent.

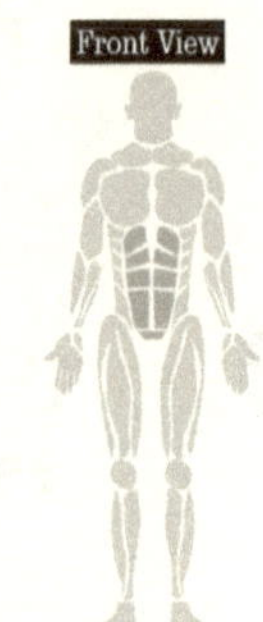

2. Place your hands on your thighs or over your chests with your forearms crossed.

3. Contract your abdominal muscles to lift your upper body off the ground to about 45°. Pause and hold at the top.

4. Keep your neck and back straight to avoid putting strain on them.

5. Slowly lower your body back to the floor and repeat the exercise.

These crunches are static, as they require you to hold the position at the top.

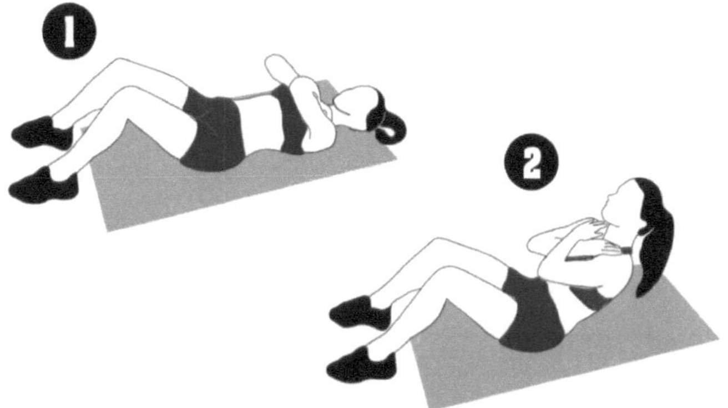
Static crunch
1
2

Russian twist

Target muscles: External obliques

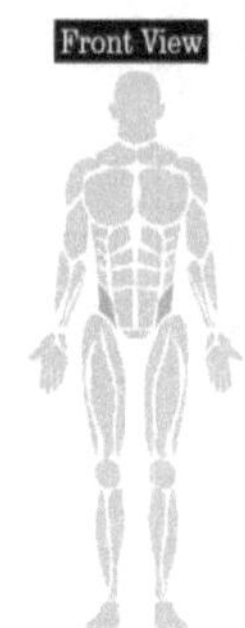

This enforces a twisting motion on the abdomen.

1. Sit with bent knees, feet on the floor for beginners or raised from the floor if you are comfortable, and lean back slightly.

2. Bring your hands together in front of you and twist your upper body from side to side, moving your hands in the same direction that you twist.

3. Exhale while you twist.

4. Hold a dumbbell to add more resistance as you get comfortable.

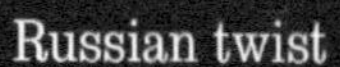
Russian twist

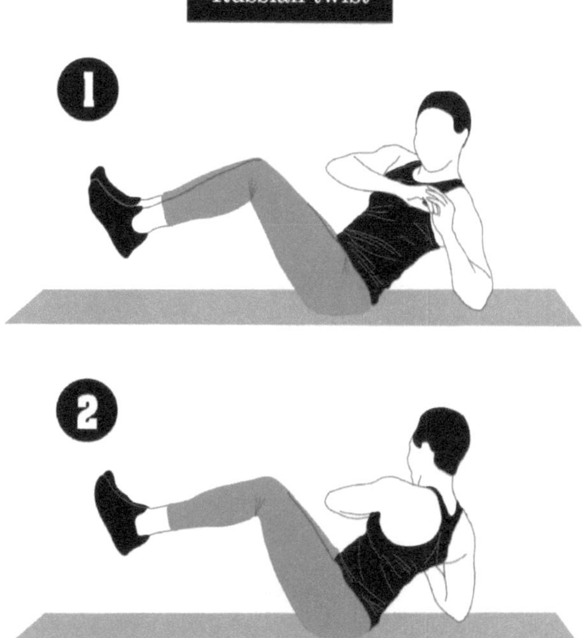

Superman

Target muscles: Erector spinae, gluteus, hamstrings

1. Lie face down on a mat with your arms outstretched, like Superman.

2. Simultaneously raise both arms and both legs, attempting to distance them from the floor.

3. Hold for 3 seconds and relax.

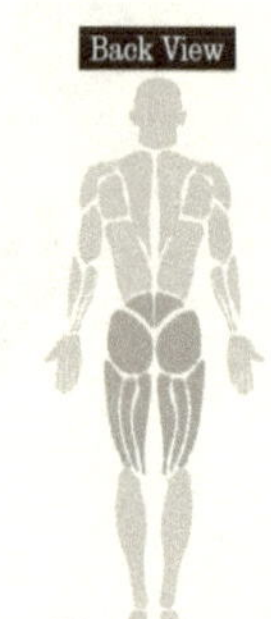

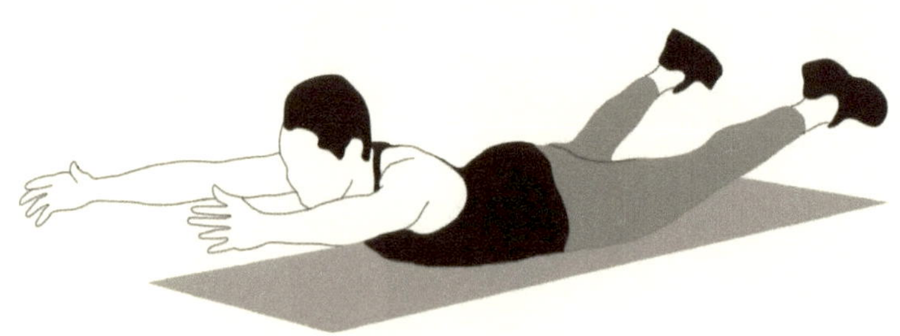

Forearm plank

Target muscles: Rectus abdominis, external obliques

1. To get into the plank position, place your forearms and toes on the floor, keeping your elbows directly under your shoulders.

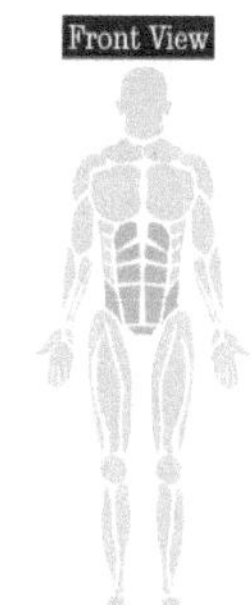

2. Contract your core muscles to solidify your body like a plank.

3. Keep your body straight from your toes to your head. Your neck should be aligned with your back and your face gazing down.

4. Hold the position for the required amount of time (as described in the next chapter).

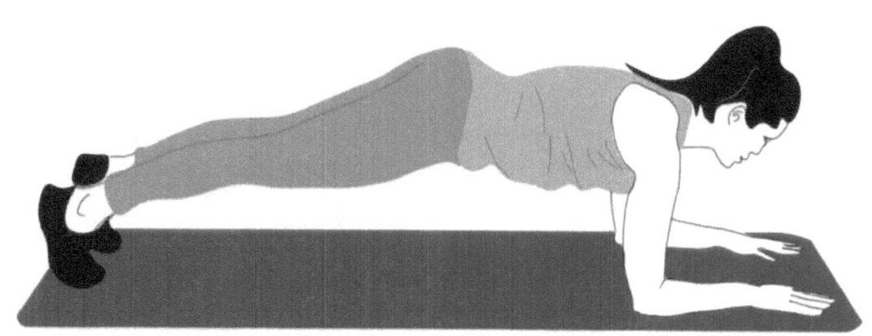

Seated shoulder dumbbell press

Target muscles: Anterior deltoid, triceps

1. While seated with your back supported, raise the dumbbells just above your shoulders, keeping your elbows bent to 90° and your palms facing forward.

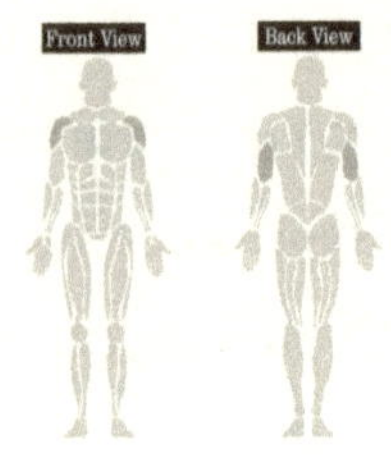

2. Exhale as you raise the weights over your head.

3. Bring them back down to shoulder level in a nicely controlled manner while inhaling.

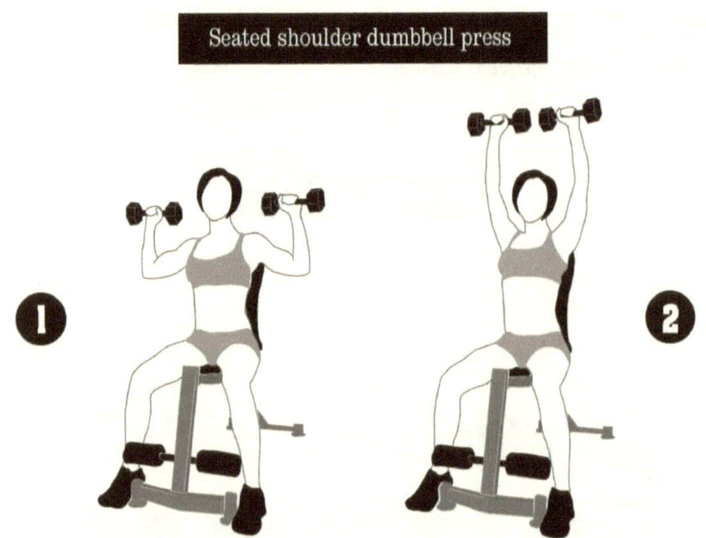

Seated cable row

Target muscles: Latissimus dorsi, rhomboids

1. On the seated row machine, sit with a straight back and your chin up.

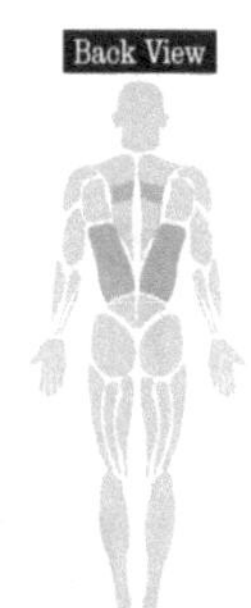

2. Lean forward and hold the handles of the bar. Pull the handles with your arms extended in front of you until you reach a 90° position between your upper body and your thighs. Stick out your chest. This is the starting position.

3. With your arms close to your torso, pull the cables back until you touch your abdominal muscles.

4. Keep the handle there for 3 seconds while exhaling.

5. Inhale as you release the cable back to the starting position.

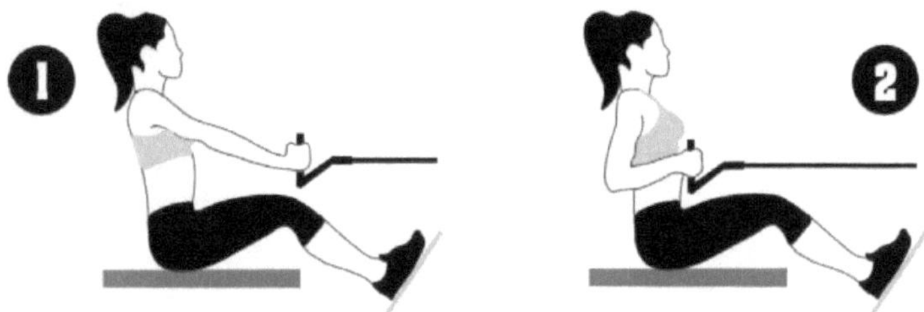

Home alternative:

This can be done on a rowing machine, as well as with resistance bands attached to your extended legs with flexed feet.

Single-arm dumbbell row

Target muscles: Latissimus dorsi

1. Place your right knee and toes on one end of a bench and stretch your right arm toward the other end. Bend over until your back is parallel to the ceiling, maintaining a natural curve in your spine.

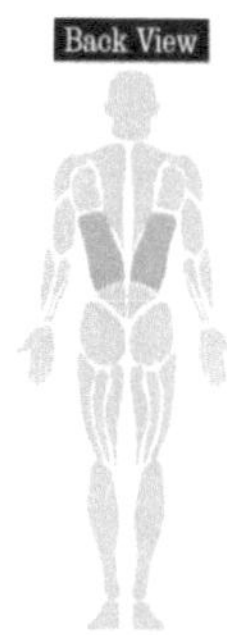

2. Extend your left leg back, keeping your foot flat on the floor.

3. With your left arm stretched, grab a dumbbell in your left hand. Your palm should be facing you.

4. Retract your shoulder blade and lift the dumbbell toward your chest by moving your elbow toward your hip and beyond. Keep your elbow close to your torso during this movement and concentrate on your latissimus dorsi.

5. Lower the weight back down. Switch sides and repeat with equal amount of reps.

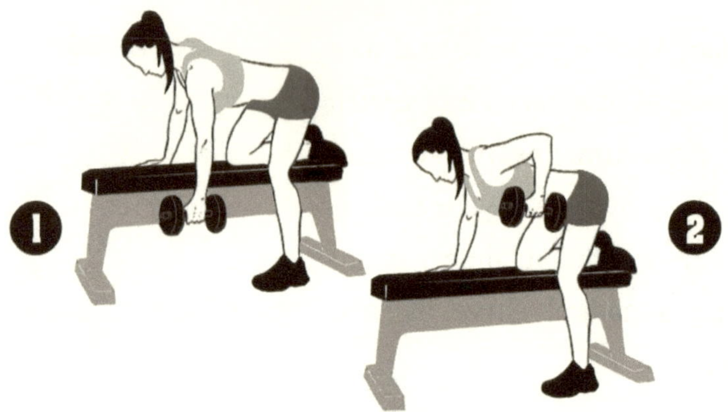
Single-arm dumbbell row
1
2

COMPOUND EXERCISES

<u>Leg press</u>

Target muscles: Quadriceps

1. While seated with your back resting on the machine pad, flex your hip at approximately 45° and your knees at about 90°.

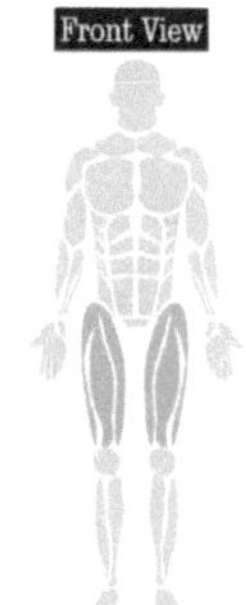

2. Place your feet flat on the plate in front of you. Do not let your knees go above the level of your toes.

3. Contract your quadriceps to move the plate forward as you extend your leg.

4. Avoid locking the knees.

5. While inhaling, bend the knees slowly back to the original position.

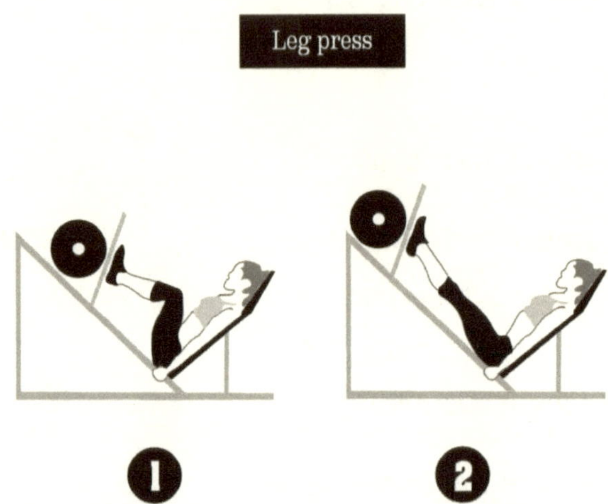

This exercise is impossible to perform without a machine. It can be replaced by a squat with two resistance bands held between the shoulders and below the feet.

Squat

Target muscles: Quadriceps, hamstrings, gluteus, core muscles

1. From a shoulder-width standing position, extend your arms in front of you for balance.

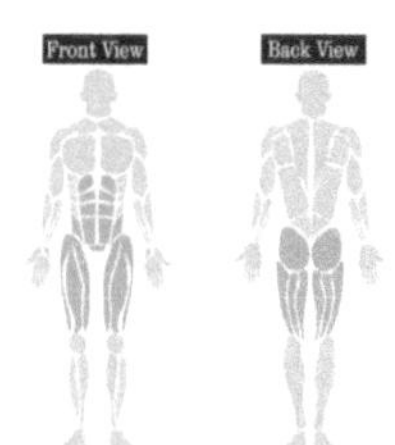

2. Lower your body to a seated position by pushing your hips backward and downward until your thighs are parallel to the floor, while maintaining a natural curve in the lower back.

3. Slowly rise back to the starting position without locking your knees. Maintain good distribution of weight between the two legs throughout.

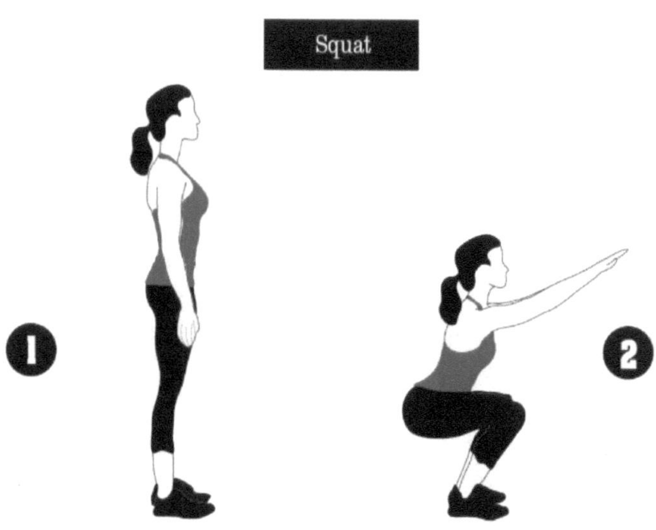

Front barbell squat

Target muscles: Quadriceps, hamstrings, gluteus, core muscles

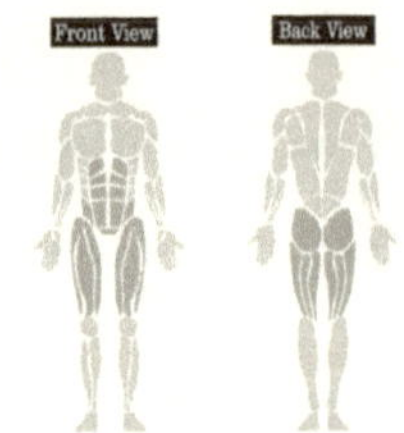

1. Walk up to the loaded bar placed on the rack at about your shoulder height and place your fingers under and around the bar with your wrist facing the ceiling. Depending on your wrist flexibility, you may find that using either two (index and middle), three (index, middle and ring), or four (index, middle, ring and pinky) fingers works best. All four fingers under the bar is ideal.

2. With your elbows facing forward and not flared out, make sure the bar is resting on your shoulders just above the level of your clavicle. Your fingers should not carry the weight of the bar, only support it.

3. Puff your chest and unrack the bar, moving a few steps back. Keep your hands at shoulder width and your feet a little wider than hip width. This is the starting position.

4. Brace your core and descend into a sitting position with your back straight and your feet flat on the ground, until your thighs are parallel to the floor.

5. Squeeze your glutes and drive through your heels as you rise back into the starting position.

6. Do the required number of reps as stated in the following chapter and safely re-rack the bar.

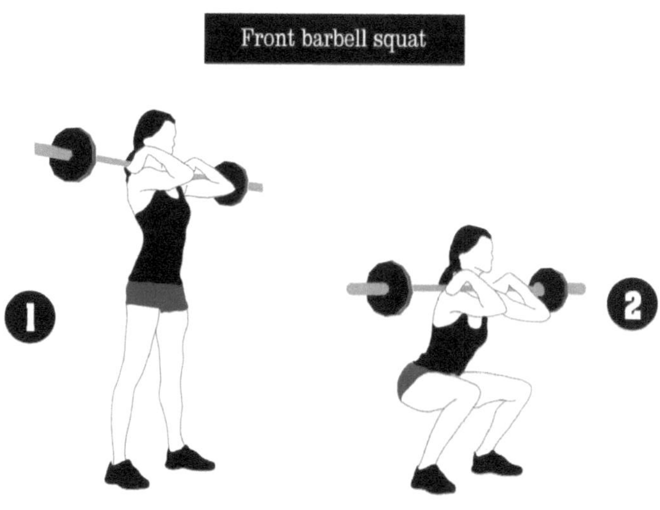

Home alternative:

Use a large loop resistance band for this exercise. Stand on the band with your feet shoulder-width apart and loop it around the top of your shoulders. Raise your arms in front of you with your elbows at a 90° angle to maintain good position and keep the band in place. Do steps 4 and 5 above.

<u>Deadlift</u>

Target muscles: Quadriceps, hamstrings, erector spinae, gluteus

1. Stand over the barbell and bend over.

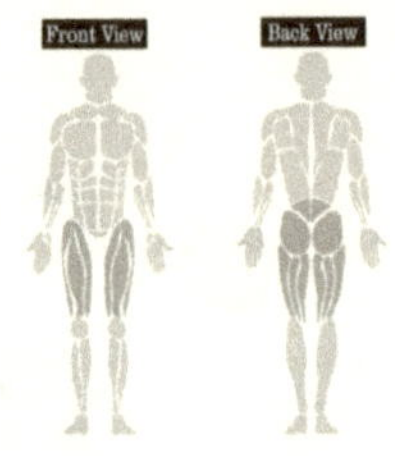

2. Place your hands shoulder-width apart on the bar. Be sure to keep your back straight.

3. Bend your knees until your shins touch the bar.

4. Lift your chest and straighten your lower back. Take a deep breath and hold it.

5. Lift the weight by standing up while exhaling slowly. Stay erect for 2 seconds.

6. Lower the weight slowly, inhaling again. Be sure to put the weight down on the floor.

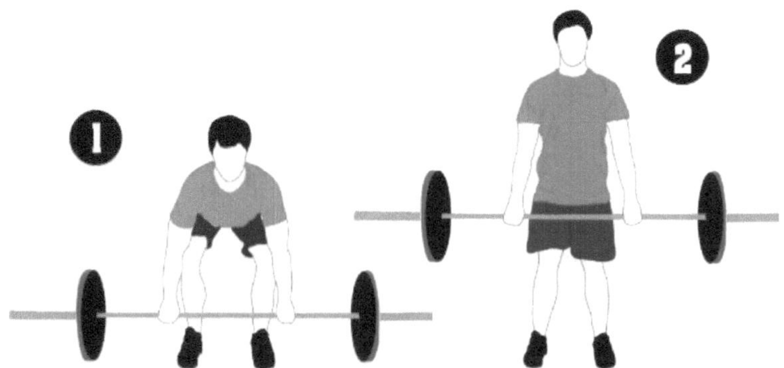

Home alternative:

This can be done at home with two dumbbells.

Semi-stiff leg deadlift

Target muscles: Hamstrings

1. Standing with your feet at hip width and your back straight, bend at your hips and grab the barbell with your arms extended. Rise up slowly as you lift the barbell off the ground and do not lock your knees. This is the starting position.

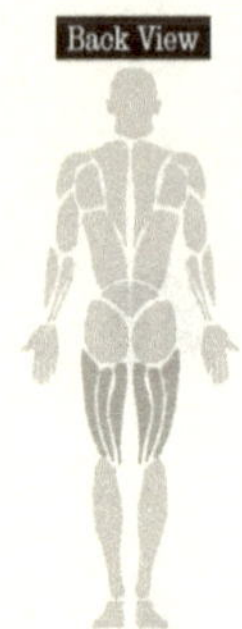

2. With the barbell in your extended arms, bend at your hips as you lower the weight to about mid-shin. You should feel a stretch in your hamstrings at this point.

3. Rise back up to the starting position and end with a slight forward hip thrust. Do not flex your knees throughout this exercise; keep them slightly bent.

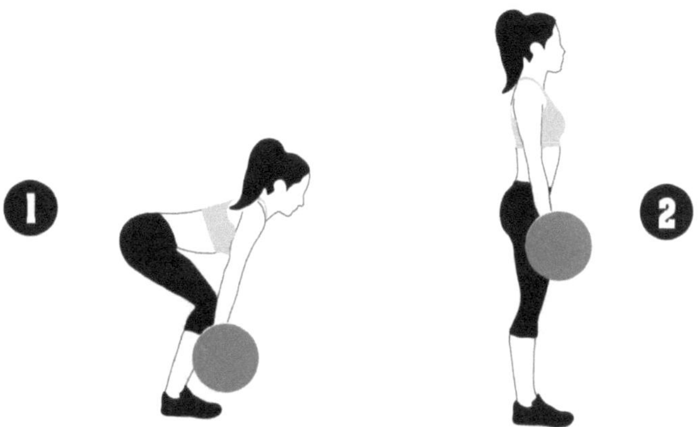
Semi-stiff leg deadlift

Static lunge

Target muscles: Quadriceps, hamstrings, gluteus

1. Start with your feet shoulder-width apart.

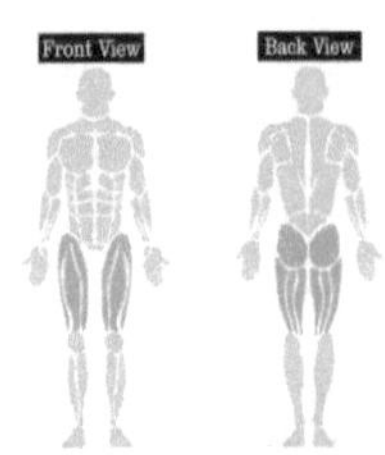

2. Take a large step forward while keeping the torso erect. This is the starting position.

3. Slowly flex your back knee until it hovers a few inches from the floor. Be careful that the front knee does not push forward past your toes.

4. Contract the quadriceps in the front leg and rise back up to the starting position.

5. Repeat movement on the other leg.

Static lunge

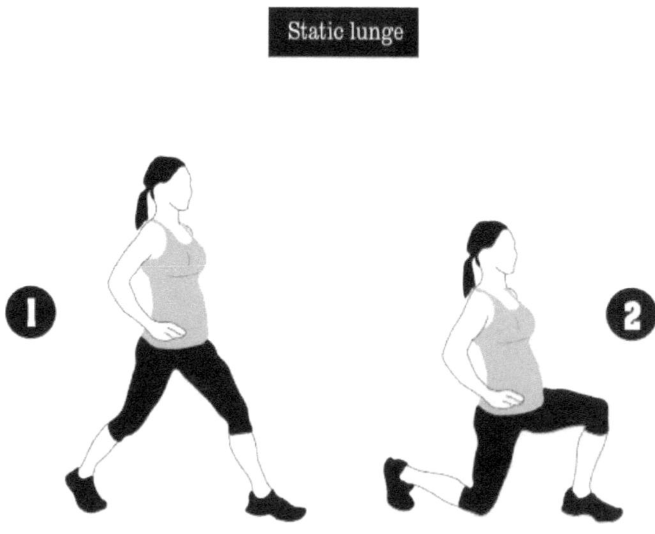

For added resistance, use dumbbells: Hold them in your hands, either in front of your chest or on either side of your body.

Walking lunge adds a dynamic aspect to this exercise, improving overall stability. This is similar to the above, except instead of returning to the starting position, you bring the back leg to meet the front leg as if you're walking. Alternate front and back legs while doing this exercise.

Incline chest dumbbell press

Target muscles: Pectoralis major (especially fibers originating from the clavicle), triceps

1. While sitting on an incline bench, grab a pair of dumbbells and hold them at the lower end of your thighs with your palms facing each other.

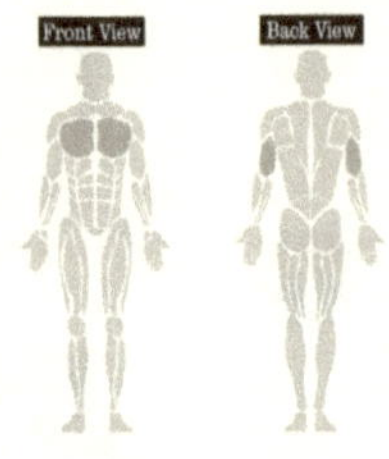

2. Use your legs to push the dumbbells up into position by your outer chest. Retract your scapula and lay back on the bench, maintaining an arch in your back and keeping your sacrum and head firmly placed on the bench. Your elbows should be flexed to about 45°. This is the starting position.

3. Press the dumbbells up with your palms facing forward without locking the elbows.

4. Bring the weights down until they just touch your outer chest without flaring your elbows.

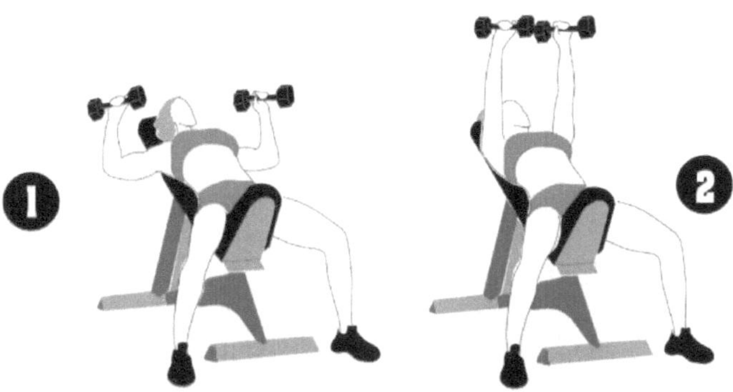

Note: Return back to sitting position and gently lower weights to your thighs and then to the floor when you have completed this exercise.

Flat barbell bench press

Target muscles: Triceps, pectoralis major, anterior deltoid

1. Lying on the flat bench, make a natural arch in your lower back while the barbell is above your eyes in the rack.

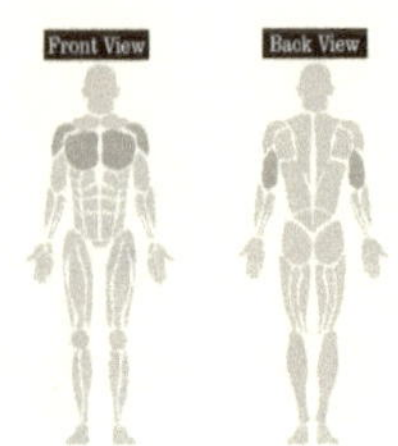

2. Grasp it and, while inhaling, bring the bar down to your chest.

3. Push the bar back up while exhaling.

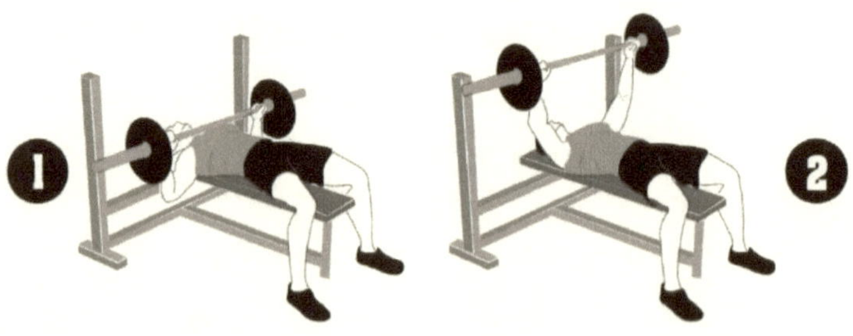

Dumbbell overhead press

Target muscles: Anterior deltoid, rotator cuff, upper trapezius

1. Stand with your feet shoulder-width apart and knees slightly bent, holding a dumbbell in each hand. Keep the muscles of the upper back tight.

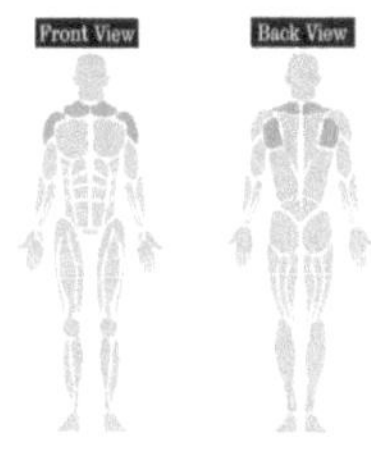

2. Raise the dumbbell to the side of your head until your upper arms are parallel to the floor and your elbows bent at 90°. Your palms should be facing forward. This is the starting position.

3. Exhale and push the dumbbells up over your head.

4. Lower the dumbbells down back to the starting position while inhaling.

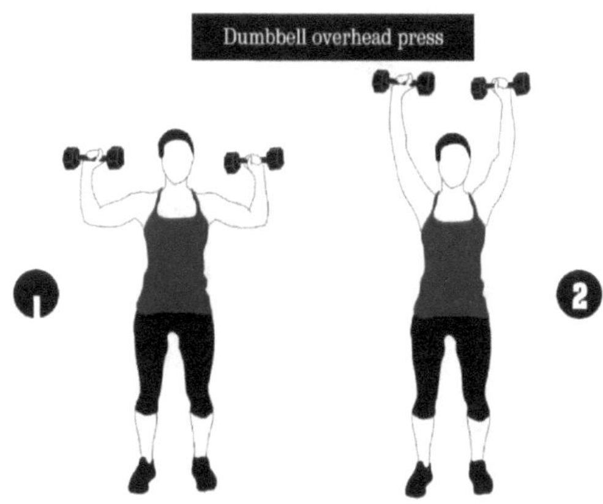

Barbell bent-over row

Target muscles: Latissimus dorsi, rhomboids, trapezius

1. In a standing with your feet hip-width apart, grab a barbell with an underhand grip keeping your hands at shoulder-width.

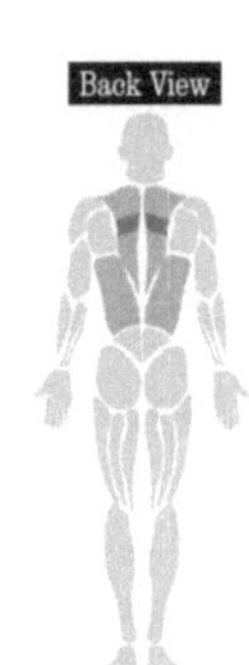

2. With a slight bend in your knees and your back straight, push your hips back until your torso is at a 45° bend or almost parallel to the floor.

3. Exhale as you bring the barbell to your midriff, and inhale as you lower it down to your knee level.

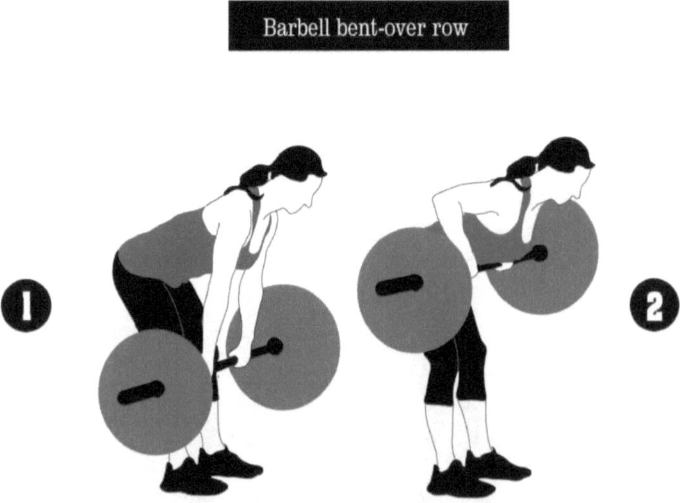

Cardio exercise

The list of what would pass as cardio exercises is endless and includes but isn't limited to walking, running (either on a treadmill or outdoors), swimming, cycling, jogging, and rowing. Exercises on a treadmill are easier to monitor, thanks to their built-in features.

As long as the selected exercise tasks your cardiorespiratory system more than usual, it works! A good way to know this is to try the 'talk test' after doing the exercise. You'll know that it's a good cardio exercise if you're unable to talk without having to pause every three to five seconds in order to catch your breath.

*"The **LAST THREE OR FOUR REPS** is what makes the muscle grow. This area of pain divides the **CHAMPION** from someone else who is not a champion. That's what most people lack, having the guts to go on and just say they'll go through the pain no matter what happens."*

— ARNOLD SCHWARZENEGGER

PART IV
WORKOUT PROGRAM

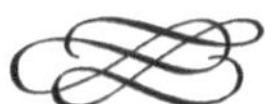

The workout program developed here follows a much-approved system of one month of endurance training, one month of strength training, and one month combining these. This enables a person over 40 to start slow, by first building their endurance. This is crucial as it prevents existing health issues from being stressed and worsening.

Furthermore, if a person suffers from chronic conditions that affect the cardiorespiratory system, it is crucial that they start slowly to adapt their heart and their breathing capacity. Health specialists recommend training cardio gradually, on a treadmill.

The workout program is designed for you to include the weights you are training with. The calculus that will enable you to personalize the weights you should be using, as well as the heart rate you should be targeting, are provided. It might be easier for you to photocopy these pages and annotate them accordingly to the week you are training.

The exercises have been detailed in the previous chapter. Be careful to bend your knees slightly in all standing positions.

THE PROGRAM

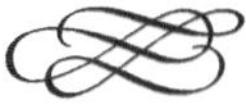

FIRST MONTH: BUILDING YOUR MUSCULAR ENDURANCE

The first month of the workout plan focuses on endurance, which requires using lighter weights and performing sets containing more repetitions (15 to 20). The weight or resistance you use should enable such sets. A field is left vacant for you to track this.

Week 1, Day 1, Lower body				
Exercise	Set x Reps	Heart rate	Weight	Notes
Leg Extension	3 x 15	55% to 60%		
Leg Press	3 x 15	55% to 60%		
Leg Curl	3 x 15	55% to 60%		
Squat	3 x 15	55% to 60%		Wide stance
Back Extension	3 x 15	55% to 60%		
Calf Raise	3 x 20	55% to 60%		
Week 1, Day 2, Upper Body				
Overhand Lat Pull Down	3 x 15	60% to 70%		Wide grip
Machine Chest Press	3 x 15	55% to 60%		Don't lock elbows
Seated Lateral Raise	3 x 15	55% to 60%		
Biceps Curl	3 x 15	55% to 60%		
Triceps Pushdown	3 x 15	55% to 60%		
Face Pull	3 x 15	55% to 60%		
Static Crunch	3 x 15	55% to 60%		3 sed hold on top
Superman	3 x 10	55% to 60%		
Forearm Plank	3 x 30 s	60% to 75%		
Week 1, Day 3, Combined				
Squat	3 x 15	55% to 60%		Narrow stance
Leg Press	3 x 15	55% to 60%		
Flat Barbell Bench Press	3 x 15	55% to 75%		
Seated Cable Row	3 x 15	55% to 60%		Close grip
Biceps Curl	3 x 15	55% to 60%		
Leg Extension	3 x 15	55% to 60%		
Triceps Extension	3 x 15	55% to 60%		
Standing Calf Raise	3 x 20	55% to 60%		
Cardio	20 min	60% to 75%		

This weekly program is to be repeated throughout the endurance month. This will adapt your nervous system and your muscular system to working out at low to moderate intensity. It also enables you to experience various levels of heart rates. This trains your cardiovascular endurance, leading to good performance during the strength month.

At the end of this endurance month, if you wish to track your progress, you are welcome to redo the Basic Fitness Assessment and compare your results.

SECOND MONTH: TRAINING MUSCULAR STRENGTH

To train muscular strength, more stress has to be put onto muscles to increase muscle tissue. As a result, more calories will be burnt, both to produce new muscle cells as well as to maintain them.

The repetitions within a set decrease as weight and resistance increase. For each exercise, it is important to identify your 1RM. This will help you understand which weight and resistance you should be using for each exercise. The weights should range between 70% and 85% of your 1RM. Heart rate should range between 60% and 75% of your age-based rate.

Week 5, Day 1, Pull			
Exercise	*Set x Reps*	*Weight*	*Notes*
Barbell Bent-over Row	3 x 12, 10, 8		Wide grip
Single-arm Dumbbell Row	3 x 12, 10, 8		
Seated Cable Row	3 x 12, 10, 8		Close grip
Supinated Lat Pulldown	3 x 12, 10, 8		Wide grip
Biceps Curl	3 x 12, 10, 8		With barbell
Single-arm Isometric Biceps Curl	3 x 12, 10, 8		
Bent-over Reverse Fly	3 x 10		
Face Pull	3 x 15		
Week 5, Day 2, Push			
Flat Barbell Bench Press	3 x 12, 10, 8		
Incline Chest Dumbbell Press	3 x 12, 10, 8		
Standing Shoulder Dumbbell Press	3 x 12, 10, 8		
Standing Lateral Raise	3 x 12		
Triceps Pushdown	3 x 12, 10, 8		With rope
Supinated Triceps Pushdown	3 x 12, 10, 8		With straight bar
Week 5, Day 3, Lower Body			
Leg Extension	3 x 12, 10, 8		Don't lock your knees
Front Barbell Squat	3 x 12, 10, 8		Wide stance
Semi-stiff Leg Deadlift	3 x 12, 10, 8		
Static Lunge	3 x 10		
Leg Press	3 x 12, 10, 8		
Back Extension	3 x 12, 10, 8		
Standing Calf Raise	3 x 20		
Static Crunch	3 x 15		3 sec hold on top
Russian Twist	3 x 10		
Forearm Plank	3 x 30 sec		

Continue this workout during the entire strength month. It is important that you track the weights that you use, increasing them when you no longer feel challenged. It would be useful to copy this workout to record the different weights you used each week.

THIRD MONTH: COMBINING ENDURANCE AND STRENGTH EXERCISES

The next month combines endurance and strength by making you perform compound exercises that activate antagonistic muscles. This advanced training will increase your heart rate; however, by now, after following the two previous months' workouts, the endurance of your cardiovascular system should have adapted. The first two endurance sets use a lighter weight, then increases in the 3rd and 4th sets, while the 5th one is again endurance with a lighter weight.

Week 9, Day 1, Chest and Back			
Exercise	*Set x Reps*	*Weight*	*Notes*
Flat Barbell Bench Press	5 x 15, 12, 10, 8, 6		
Barbell Bent-over Row	5 x 15, 12, 10, 8, 6		
Incline Chest Dumbbell Press	3 x 12, 10, 8		
Single-arm Dumbbell Row	3 x 12, 10, 8		
Cable Chest Crossover	5 x 15, 12, 10, 8, 6		
Seated Cable Row	5 x 15, 12, 10, 8, 6		
Week 9, Day 2, Deltoid, Biceps, Triceps			
Seated Shoulder Dumbbell Press	5 x 15, 12, 10, 8, 6		
Seated Lateral Raise	5 x 15, 12, 10, 8, 6		
Biceps Curl (with Barbell)	3 x 12, 10, 8		
Single-arm Isometric Biceps Curl	3 x 12, 10, 8		
One-arm Overhead Triceps Extension	3 x 12, 10, 8		With rope
Supinated Triceps Pushdown	3 x 12, 10, 8		
Face Pull	3 x 15		
Cardio	20 min		
Week 9, Day 3, Lower Body			
Leg Extension	3 x 15		
Walking Lunge	3 x 40 steps		Added weight optional
Deadlift	4 x 10, 8, 6, 4		
Semi-stiff Leg Deadlift	3 x 12, 10, 8		
Leg Curl	3 x 15		
Seated Calf Raise	3 x 15		
Static Crunch	3 x 20		2 sec hold on top
Russian Twist	3 x 30 sec		
Forearm Plank	3 x 1 min		

Continue this for the rest of the third month. By now, you should have a good understanding of the type of workout that helps you achieve your physical goal.

OUT OF TRAINING VARIABLES

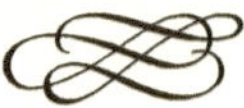

One detail you won't see on Instagram training montages is just how much of your progress depends on what you're doing outside of the gym. We're going to briefly look at these factors, why they matter, and how you should approach them.

If you're not progressing or you're struggling with your workouts, you need to evaluate and be honest with yourself about **your** habits. This is where the main results come from, so if you're skipping out on these areas, you're only cheating yourself out of better results.

NUTRITION

I've talked about nutrition already, but know that it's the driving force behind your results. If you're 80% consistent, you're going to get 80% results. And that's a lot of results to be missing out on. Before you complain about programs or your lack of results, always look at your diet.

SLEEP

If you're not sleeping eight or more hours a night, you're missing out on results. Changes here affect your hormones and thus how your body recovers, repairs, and grows.

Sleep quality is also important and there are a few ways you can help improve both the quality and quantity of your sleep:

- Cut out caffeine seven hours before bed.
- Reduce screen time in the hour before bed.
- Get plenty of sunlight during the day.
- Try to get a little bit of exercise in before bed to tire yourself out.
- Do some relaxing stretching or reading before bed.
- Make sure your room is as dark, cool, and quiet as possible.

These help you make the right choices about when to sleep and will also improve the quality of your sleep. The results can really show in your performance.

HYDRATION

Drink your water! It's a cornerstone of life itself, so you'll need to focus on keeping water nearby. If you keep a full water bottle on you at all times, your body is going to hydrate itself by habit.

You should also make sure you're getting plenty of electrolytes, which are minerals that help hydration and support muscle function—specifically, magnesium, potassium, calcium, and sodium. These should be in your diet, and you can get them in electrolyte drinks or mixes for better hydration and results.

RELAXATION AND STRESS MANAGEMENT

Stress reduces your results, suppresses your growth hormones, and is terrible for your mental health.

Spend some time actively relaxing. Schedule in activities where you can completely switch off and let your brain disengage. These are great for helping you recover from exercise, but also from life itself, and the results you see from managing them will be significant across all areas of your life.

You'll want to focus on things like reading, stretching, family time, a favorite hobby, whatever. The idea is to just **not stress**, on purpose, for a few hours a week. This reduces the risk of mood disorders like depression, improves sleep quality, and provides the perfect environment for muscle repair and growth.

CONCLUSION: KEEP AT IT!

And that about does it—everything you need to know to make your own strength training journey a success, even in your 40s and beyond. The education and guidance shared here is something you can, and should, come back to regularly, but the really important part is **doing**. I can tell you what to do, but you're the one who's going to need to make those choices, eat those foods, and put in those reps when you're training.

The beauty of all this is that, for most people, it's one of the most interesting and enjoyable ways of getting into shape. Strength training is popular not only because it's effective, but because the clear and measurable progress over time can become really enjoyable and addictive. Once you get that ball rolling, you might find it's actually no effort at all to keep up with it, but rather just a new hobby you've developed a love for.

That's how it got me, and I know that many people who never saw themselves as the "pumping iron" type found the reality of weight training to be so much better than they'd anticipated!

The kind of misgivings people have about strength training, and especially for those training over 40, are just that: ideas and expectations that disappear when they try the real thing. Building this habit is one of the best things I've ever done with my life—it's brought me a career, dozens of new friends, and a body I am happy with for the first time in my life. *Is it any wonder I recommend it so highly?*

All you need to do is get that ball rolling and keep showing up: you don't have to crush every session, you don't have to be the world's strongest man or woman, and you don't have to live up to anyone's expectations but your own. Consistency is your strongest weapon, and you can start **right now** if you give yourself the chance.

RESOURCES

Bortz, W. M. (1982). Disuse and Aging, *Journal of the American Medical Association* 248 (10), 1203–1208.

Harris, D. V. and Harris, B. L. (1984). *The Athlete's Guide to Sports Psychology: Mental Skills for Physical People.* Ann Arbor, MI, University of Michigan.

Bortz, W. M. (2007). *We Live Too Short and Die Too Long: How to Achieve and Enjoy Your Natural 100-Year-Plus Life Span.* New York, SelectBooks.

Sheldon, W. H., Stevens, S. S., and Tucker, W. B. (1940). *The Varieties of Human Physique.* New York, Harper.

Balady, G. J. (2000). *ACSM's Guidelines for Exercise Testing and Prescription* (6th edition). Philadelphia-London, Lippincott Williams & Wilkins, American College of Sports Medicine.

Gastelu, D. and Hatfield, F. C. (2019). *Sports Nutrition* (5th edition). Carpinteria, CA: International Sports Science Association.

Hatfield, F. C. (2019). *Fitness: The Complete Guide* (9th edition). Carpinteria, CA: International Sports Science Association.

ONLINE RESOURCES:

Wolff's law:

https://en.wikipedia.org/wiki/Wolff%27s_law

Identify your Body Type:

https://www.bodybuilding.com/fun/becker3.htm

Target Heart Rate:

https://www.heart.org/en/healthy-living/fitness/fitness-basics/target-heart-rates

Borg Rating of Perceived Exertion: Revised Scale:

https://www.heartonline.org.au/media/DRL/Rating_of_perceived_exertion_-_Borg_scale.pdf